Clinical Integrability

Clinical Integrability

A Grammar of Subjective Reality,
Sequence, and Change

The DDSRF Model

Dual-Domain Subjective Reality Formation

Shiraz Mamedov

First edition, 2026.

ISBN (paperback): 979-8-9965155-0-9
ISBN (ebook): 979-8-9965155-1-6

Published by DDSRF

Professional scope

This book is a professional and educational text for clinicians, supervisors, teachers, advanced students, and researchers. It is not a self-help manual, a diagnostic system, a treatment protocol, or a substitute for psychiatric assessment, crisis care, clinical supervision, informed clinical judgment, or the clinical contract. DDSRF helps clinicians read the conditions under which an intervention becomes clinically usable; it does not replace specialized care for psychosis, acute suicide risk, severe dissociation, medically unstable eating disorders, bipolar episodes, or other high-risk states.

Clinical material

Clinical examples and vignettes are illustrative. Identifying details have been altered, composited, or constructed to protect confidentiality. They are not presented as case reports unless explicitly stated.

For clinicians who keep listening.

Contents

FROM THE AUTHOR

Why I am letting this go to print

You are holding a book whose author put off writing this one page for a long time.

Every piece of work has a last bridge. The text is assembled, the terms are settled, the figures hold — and one movement remains: to let go. I stood at that bridge longer than I would like to admit. What held me was not doubt about the logic. It was two fears, and both were about me, not about the theory. The first: that I was releasing a private way of seeing — persuasive only as far as its author is persuasive — and calling it knowledge. The second I could not name for a long time without striking a pose, because it is smaller and more shameful: that the work might turn out to be alive, and then I would be the one asked to answer for it, when I am used to being the one who asks.

I understood late that I was weighing the wrong question at the bridge. I kept asking whether the theory was needed. The question I owed myself was whether I was ready to stop being its only reader. As long as a work goes unpublished, its author keeps a monopoly on reading it correctly. That is comfortable, and it is quietly dishonest: what is never released can be neither tested, nor corrected, nor even properly refuted. It stays with its author. Only by crossing the bridge does it cease to be him and become knowledge.

What finally decided me was a sober thought about the cost of being wrong. Were this book a protocol — *do this to the patient* — I would have no right to publish without full empirical proof, because the price of unproven elegance would be someone else's suffering. But DDSRF is built otherwise, and deliberately so. It is not a school of therapy, not a diagnostic system, not a treatment protocol. It is a language — a grammar for discerning, before you intervene, whether the next move can become part of another person's experience.

And a language is not "wrong" in the way an instruction can be wrong. It can turn out to be barren — but a barren language is taken up reluctantly, and that is not a frightening death. The worst that can befall this book is to go unnoticed. The worst that can befall my silence is that a distinction which might one day let you see your own patient more clearly simply never reaches you.

So I give you this work as a working hypothesis, not a verdict — and I have tried nowhere to pass off as proven what is not yet proven. Nor have I hidden the conditions under which the theory should be judged to have failed: where its distinctions must agree across different observers, and where it is more honest for it to fall silent. I would rather you read me against myself than after myself. An attentive reader's disagreement does the theory more good than an inattentive one's assent.

What remains is to admit the quietest thing. One does not cross the bridge out of certainty of being right. One crosses when one understands that the worth of a theory lies not in whether it is right, but in whether it lets others see what was invisible before. On this side of the river that cannot be checked. It is learned only after letting go.

I have crossed. Not from confidence, and not from pride — to hold on any longer would have dressed caution up as virtue, and that would have been cowardice. What comes of this language now depends not on me, but on what you are able to discern with it — at the chair, in the silence between words, where being technically right still guarantees nothing.

— Sh. M.

Introduction

This book is organized in two registers. The Main Text is read sequentially, like any theoretical-clinical text; the Method Atlas, placed after the twelve chapters, is its working continuation in a different genre. The book has twelve chapters and eleven appendices. Together they present the same material in two registers: the chapter explains, the appendix serves as support during the work. A chapter should be read in sequence; an appendix should be opened when the chapter points to it.

The book is written for the practicing clinician. The reader assumed here is a working therapist — not necessarily of many years, but already seeing clients; a supervisor; a teacher in clinical training. Secondarily it is written for researchers who need to distinguish what in DDSRF is already described from what remains hypothesis. It is not written as popular reading about psychotherapy and does not try to be; it contains no simplifications for a general audience and no psychoeducational register. Self-help is a separate genre with its own responsibilities, and this book does not belong to it.

The book offers one way of hearing the clinical moment — a grammar that a clinician of any school can use. It is not a new school of therapy, not a diagnostic system, and not a protocol. DDSRF has no techniques of its own; it does not replace the decision about what to do in the room — that remains with the approach you work from. It helps with something else: seeing why an action that is right in content may fail to land today, while two weeks later the same action lands and works. That is the subject of the first chapter, where the model's full promise unfolds; here it is enough to say that the book is about the conditions of fit, not about the rightness of technique.

The Main Text and the Method Atlas are written to work together. The chapters are a sequential learning spiral: each concept rests on the previous one, and reading the chapters out of order is not recommended. The Atlas is built differently: it is not read straight through from A to K. It is better opened as the chapters proceed — each chapter, at the right moment, points to the corresponding appendix, and at those moments the Atlas opens as working support rather than as a separate textbook. A special case is Appendix A, the DDSRF Case Card: it draws the whole apparatus onto a single page of case formulation, and it is useful to keep at hand throughout the reading. The remaining appendices are best opened when the corresponding chapter refers to them.

And one more thing — a short contract. The book does not ask you to change your school, learn a new protocol, or believe in a new system. It offers one additional question alongside the one you already ask of every intervention: not "is this right," but "can this land now." If that question proves useful, the book has done its work. If at some point it does not prove useful, that too matters: that is where the limit of the language runs. The model is designed to be revisable and testable, not final; how it limits itself and where it is obliged to fall silent is the subject of the last, twelfth chapter. Beyond this — the clinical scene with which everything begins.

Part I

The Problem and the Architecture

Chapter 1. Premature Rightness

1.1. A scene any experienced therapist recognizes

Imagine a session that was going very well.

The client — a woman of about forty, two years into the work — has left a marriage she had for many years lived as a zone of silent suppression. Today, for the first time, she said it in words, without reservations or softening. She was crying — not from grief but from relief. The therapist heard it precisely. And at what seemed the right moment said: "It sounds as if for many years you wouldn't let yourself know how bad it was for you there."

It was a right interpretation. It had been prepared by all the preceding work. The tone was calm, without pressure. And yet — the client fell silent. For a few seconds she looked out the window. Then she said, "Yes, probably," and began to talk about something else entirely, something everyday. A week later she came in low and said she felt she was "moving in the wrong direction." Another week later she asked whether it might be worth taking a break.

The therapist went over everything he could in his mind. The interpretation was not aggressive. It did not intrude. It named what the client had almost said herself. Technically it was a clean, careful step. And it was precisely after it that the closing-down occurred.

This scene is known to everyone who has worked for long. Each school has its own words for it. Psychoanalysis will speak of a premature interpretation, of unreadiness to work with this affect, of the analyst running ahead of the transference. A cognitive-behavioral therapist will think of moving too quickly through the protocol, of low readiness to change, of a poor fit between the intervention and the current stage. An ACT practitioner will see fusion with self-criticism, activated by the named loss. A trauma therapist will feel that the client has left the window of tolerance. A Gestalt therapist will speak of an interruption of contact. A systemic therapist — that the therapist named what, in the client's family, it was forbidden to name.

Each of these explanations works inside its own school. And each speaks, in essence, of one and the same thing — but in different languages. Between the languages, what is lost is the common element that explains why such a situation recurs for clinicians of all schools, for the experienced and the beginning alike, in different contexts and with different clients.

That common element is the subject of this book.

1.2. A name for a shared clinical pain

I propose to call this situation premature rightness. The word "premature" is old; psychoanalysts will recognize it. The word "rightness" is neutral, not tied to any school. Together they name a precise clinical assembly: an intervention that was right in content and wrong for the moment.

What does "right in content" mean? It means that if the client could take it in, it would be accurate for them. It names what is there. It rests on what is already visible. It moves in the right direction. Technically it is not an error.

What does "wrong for the moment" mean? It means that the client's current subjective reality cannot include it. Not understand it — include it. The client in the example above could understand perfectly well. She was educated, reflective, long in the work. Understanding was not blocked. What was blocked was integration — what separates "I heard this" from "this is now part of how I experience myself."

The distinction between understanding and integration is one of the load-bearing distinctions of this book. We will return to it in Chapter 4. For now it matters to see that the technically right interpretation in this scene met not a failure to understand but an organization of experience that could not hold it. The client had just said aloud, for the first time, what she had for years not let herself know. Her assembly of reality at that moment was occupied with holding the very fact of the utterance. Any additional load — even an accurate and supportive one — exceeded the capacity. The closing-down was not resistance. It was the work of a system protecting its fragile new coherence.

This formulation is worth saying once more. A closing-down after a right intervention is not resistance and not the client's fault. It is the normal work of a system protecting its current wholeness from overload.

And here too — a symmetrical observation, without which the book would be incomplete. If the therapist, seeing the client's tears, had said nothing and done nothing beyond staying with her, that too could have been right. Not out of caution and not out of fear of interpreting. But out of a reading of the moment, in which the main event had already happened — the client had spoken for the first time. No interpretation could strengthen it. Any interpretation could take the authorship of that moment from the client and hand it to the therapist.

Premature rightness does not mean the therapist should have stayed silent. It means that at this moment any verbal addition beyond the most minimal was a load, not a help. The therapist could have said a single word — "yes," or the client's name, or simply nodded and stayed in the breath beside her. That would have been enough. The system could not include more.

The distinction between a "right interpretation" and "a response fit for the moment" is the very gap in which premature rightness lives. And in this gap all clinicians spend a significant part of their working time.

1.3. Why the school explanations are not enough

If each school already has its own explanation of this situation, why is another needed?

Because the school explanations work from inside the school and translate poorly into one another. A psychoanalyst speaking of a premature interpretation and a CBT therapist speaking of low readiness to change are describing the same clinical event — but their descriptions do not converge into a common picture. When the two sit in one supervision and discuss one case, they must either switch to the language of one of the schools or talk in parallel. They have no common operational language for the event itself.

This is not an academic problem. It is a practical one. A therapist trained by a psychoanalyst and working in an institution with CBT protocols must switch between languages within a single session. A supervisor whose group holds clinicians of different schools cannot rely on a common description of the moment and is forced to work through metaphors. A graduate student reading the literature of different traditions sees that one and the same clinical situation is called by different names, and cannot tell whether these names refer to the same thing or to different things.

There is a more serious problem too. School explanations tend to shift blame. The psychoanalytic language — onto the client's resistance or the analyst's own error. The CBT language — onto "low motivation" or "poor fit." The ACT language — onto fusion. The trauma language — onto dysregulation. Each of these names points to something real, but each at the same time makes something narrow. Resistance is about the client. Dysregulation is about the body. Fusion is about avoidance processes. All these names are partial, and none describes the structure of the moment itself — why precisely this intervention at precisely this moment turned out incompatible with precisely this state of the assembly of experience.

School explanations also tend toward one of two typical errors: they either over-individualize (it is all about this particular client and their history) or over-generalize (it is the work of a defense mechanism that operates in everyone). The first error loses the common. The second loses the particular. Between them falls what needs to be seen: the common structure of the moment, realized concretely in this client.

DDSRF offers a description of that common structure. Not instead of the school languages, but a level below them — as a grammar on which these languages can be reconciled. In this grammar premature rightness has a precise place, and it can be shown.

1.4. Where premature rightness lives

Premature rightness lives in the gap between two characteristics of an intervention: its rightness in content and its fit for the moment.

Rightness in content is determined inside the school. What counts as a right interpretation is decided by psychoanalytic theory. What counts as a successful behavioral experiment is decided by the CBT frame, the process-based case formulation, or a particular therapeutic protocol. What counts as an apt paradoxical intervention is decided by systemic theory. Each school has its own criteria of rightness, and DDSRF does not interfere with them.

Fit for the moment is determined at another level. It depends not on the theory of a school but on the current state of the client's subjective reality — on whether their assembly of experience can include this intervention without closing-down, fragmentation, or pseudo-agreement. This fit is not determined by any of the schools within their own apparatus. It is determined by what DDSRF calls integrative capacity — the throughput of the current assembly for new material.

From this follows a simple but important thing. An intervention can be at once right in content and unfit for the moment. Not despite its rightness, but independently of it. These two characteristics live on different axes. And it is their discrepancy that creates premature rightness.

This gives us a clinical definition that can be used in the work:

> Premature rightness is a discrepancy between the rightness of an intervention in content and its fit for the moment, in which the client's system cannot integrate the intervention because its integrative capacity at that moment is lower than the load of the intervention requires.

This definition does several things. It separates the problem of fit from the problem of rightness — freeing the therapist from the false dichotomy "either I did the right or the wrong thing." It introduces the notion of load, to which we will return in Chapter 4. It introduces the notion of integrative capacity — a working category of the whole book. And it makes premature rightness not a moral category but a structural one.

A therapist who has made a premature-right intervention has not "erred" in the human sense. He has performed a clinically right action that at this moment turned out unsuited to the current state of the assembly. These are different positions, and they hold the whole ethics of the book. The counter-example in DDSRF is not a story about a therapist at fault. It is a story about a clinical situation in which the fit between load and capacity did not come about — and which can be read more precisely.

1.5. The symmetrical error: perpetual stabilization

If DDSRF spoke only of premature rightness, it would be a theory of caution. A theory of “don’t rush,” “give the client time,” “don’t intrude.” There is already plenty of that in the clinical literature, and it generates a clinical problem of its own.

The symmetrical error of premature rightness is **perpetual stabilization**.

This is the situation in which a therapist, trained (often rightly) to fear overloading the client, never creates the conditions for a counter-experience. Each time the possibility of something new appears in the work, the therapist regulates, supports, normalizes, returns to the safe zone. The sessions go well. The client feels understood and protected. The alliance is strong. There are no complaints. But after a year, after two, after four — the client’s reality is the same. What has changed is their capacity to experience it inside therapy. What has not changed is how it is assembled outside.

Perpetual stabilization is a clinical error of the same rank as premature rightness. It is simply less visible. A premature intervention causes closing-down, and that can be seen. Perpetual stabilization causes nothing acute — and that is precisely why it can be done for years without notice. Especially in approaches that place alliance or regulation above all else, and from which the notion has dropped away that an experience not matching the habitual assembly is necessary.

An important caveat belongs here. There are clinical cases where stabilization is the work. States of deep dysregulation, severe trauma presentations, early phases of treatment, periods of crisis — in these situations, building stable regulation does not precede therapy, it is therapy. DDSRF does not deny this. Moreover, in the scale of Cα integration modes (Chapter 5) there is a stabilizing mode, described as a full mode, not a deficient one.

The distinction between clinically indicated stabilization and perpetual stabilization as an error comes down to one thing: the first creates the conditions for a future counter-experience, the second makes it impossible. The first increases integrative capacity. The second preserves it unchanged. From the outside, in the short term, they look alike. They can be told apart only by what happens to the system’s capacity over time.

This symmetrical naming of two errors — premature rightness and perpetual stabilization — is one of the load-bearing ethical constructions of the book. DDSRF is not a theory of caution. Nor a theory of courage. It is a theory of fit — between load and capacity, between moment and intervention, between what is introduced and what can be taken in.

Sometimes the fit means slowing down. Sometimes it means stepping outside the habitual zone. Sometimes silence that would be offensive in another moment. Sometimes a sentence that in another moment would be premature. The decision depends not on a theoretical preference for one over the other but on a reading of the current state of the assembly.

1.6. Why this is not a question of experience

One might think that premature rightness is a beginner's disease, and that it passes with experience. It does not.

The experienced clinician does indeed make large premature interventions less often. They have learned to feel the moment, to recognize the signs of readiness, to hold a pause. But experience does not abolish premature rightness. It shifts it to a finer level.

The beginning therapist makes a premature interpretation where even a textbook would show it is early. The experienced one makes it where the textbook would not show it, but where the client's system is not yet ready. The experienced therapist has their own blind spot: they have learned to trust their sense of the moment, and sometimes that sense is calibrated to a particular type of client or a particular configuration of experience. With a different configuration it can err, and experience by itself gives no protection — on the contrary, it can give false confidence.

There is another form of premature rightness specific to the experienced. It is a technically flawless action performed in the moment of the therapist's own counter-load. An experienced clinician who cannot withstand helplessness may make an entirely correct intervention precisely in order to step out of the helplessness. The intervention will be accurate. But its source is not a reading of the client; it is the therapist's own load, which they could not hold. The client senses this. Not consciously. But an intervention made out of an unheld counter-load lands differently than one made out of a reading of the moment. More often than not it turns out to be premature — regardless of how right it is in content.

We will return to this side of the matter in Chapter 4, when we speak of integrability as a dyadic construct: an intervention is fit only if the client, the therapist, and the field between them can hold it. For now it is enough to say that premature rightness is not only, and not so much, an error in reading the client. It is an error in reading the system of three — client, therapist, and field. And experience protects against the first component better than against the other two.

1.7. Where we go next

Premature rightness has been named. What is needed next is a language in which it can be seen in the work.

That language does not arise all at once. It is built gradually — through a series of distinctions, each answering its own question. What does the client's "current subjective reality" mean? What does "integrative capacity" mean? What modes of assembly are there, and how are they told apart? What is the "reality weight" of an experience, and why does rational agreement with an alternative not change reality? Which layer of the system currently holds the veto on the next step? What is a counter-experience, and how does it differ from insight?

Each of these questions is a separate chapter. All of them are needed for premature rightness to turn from a general observation into a working category usable in a real session.

Before we go further, one more thing is needed — to cut away what DDSRF does not do. Without this, the language we are building could quickly turn into yet another doctrine that explains everything. That is the work of Chapter 2.

And earlier still — a short closing scene.

The same case. Three weeks after the closing-down, the client returned to the theme herself. Without invitation, without the therapist's question. She said: "I've been thinking about what you said back then. I couldn't hear it. I wasn't ready. But I've been thinking." That was the moment for which this whole book is needed. The client did not reject the interpretation. She did not accept it at once. She held it in an unintegrated form for three weeks, went through her own cycle, and only then did the interpretation become part of her assembly. The therapist, at that moment, said nothing superfluous. He said: “Yes.” And they began the next step.

Between “did not land” and “landed” lies not a failure. Between them lies the work of integration, which cannot be hurried but can be understood. The rest of the book is devoted to that work.

Chapter 2. What DDSRF Claims and What It Does Not

2.1. Why a theory needs boundaries

There is a simple clinical law: a theory that explains everything helps with nothing. The wider its reach, the less it discriminates. The more precisely defined its zone of work, the more it gives within that zone.

With DDSRF this is especially worth saying at the very start. Because a theory that names the general structure of the clinical moment faces a natural temptation to spread further — onto a typology of clients, a classification of disorders, universal recommendations, a philosophy of therapy in general. Each of these extensions looks harmless from the inside. Together they turn a working category into yet another large system that explains everything and is therefore of use for nothing.

This chapter exists to set the boundaries in advance. First — the four claims on which DDSRF rests. Then — the five places where one is usually tempted to extend it, and why that must not be done. At the end — a practical criterion of compatibility with schools, because without that criterion the theory quickly turns into an ideology.

2.2. The four claims on which DDSRF rests

First. There is a general clinical event recognized by clinicians of all schools: an action right in content does not, at a given moment, land; or, symmetrically, the absence of action where a new experience is needed leaves the system in stable insensitivity. This event has no single name in the existing literature — each school names it in its own way. DDSRF offers a common working category for it: a lack of fit between the load of an intervention and the integrative capacity of the system (client, therapist, and the field between them).

This claim is operational, not philosophical. It does not require the reader to accept any metapsychology. It says: if you practice and have met the situation described in Chapter 1, you have working access to what is being discussed. What follows is a question of whether that recognition can be turned into a differentiable reading.

Second. The client's subjective reality is assembled, not reflected. This means: what is real for the client at a given moment — world, other, body, time, action — is not a passive reception of impressions but an active organization of experience that maintains its own coherence. This assembly has layers (body, the field of the other, narrative, predictive activity, thresholds of coherence, early calibration, context), and there is an operator that binds them into a single lived whole.

This claim is compatible with many theoretical frames — with predictive processing, with the intersubjective tradition, with constructivist approaches, with phenomenological psychiatry. DDSRF is not tied to any one of them as a foundation. It uses the notion of assembly as a working one: it is needed to explain why the same content of an intervention yields different clinical results at different moments in the same client. Without the notion of assembly, that difference would have to be explained by circumstance, mood, or luck. With the notion of assembly, it becomes readable.

Third. Change in therapy happens not through understanding but through integration. These are two different levels. To understand is to include in semantic content. To integrate is to change how the assembly organizes the next experience. Between them may lie a week, may lie a year, may lie a whole life. No theory that identifies these two levels can explain the gap between "the client understood everything" and "nothing changed."

DDSRF makes this distinction load-bearing. From it follows an operational definition of a fit intervention: an intervention fit at a given moment is one the system can integrate without closing down, without fragmenting, and without simulating agreement. This definition is empty until we have instruments for reading the state of the assembly. Those instruments — Cα modes, reality weight, the dominant constraint, the minimal counter-experience — are given in the following chapters. For now it matters to fix that the definition of integrability is descriptive, not normative. DDSRF does not say what should be integrated. It says what can be integrated now.

Fourth. The therapist is part of the system that reads and changes the client's subjective reality, not an outside observer. This means something concrete: an intervention is fit only when three elements can hold it, not one. The client, with their current assembly. The therapist, with their own load and capacity. The field S(t) between them. If the therapist cannot hold their own shame, helplessness, or urge to rescue, the field breaks from the therapist's side, and a technically correct intervention ceases to be fit — regardless of what happens with the client.

This claim is not often formulated in the clinical literature as structural rather than sentimental. DDSRF makes it one of its load-bearing supports. From it follows that the therapist's counter-load is not part of their supervisory work, left off the clinical stage. It is part of the clinical reading of the moment itself. Chapter 4, where the notions of load and capacity are introduced, unfolds this point into a working category.

These four claims are enough for DDSRF to have a subject. It claims nothing more.

2.3. The five places where DDSRF does not work

Now — the reverse side. Each claim in 2.2 corresponds to something. And each has a boundary beyond which DDSRF loses its force. These boundaries are important to name, because it is just beyond them that a working category begins to turn into an ideology.

DDSRF is not a diagnostic system. The book will have concepts — configurations, dominant layers, Cα modes. The temptation to use them as diagnostic categories — to call a client a "shame configuration," a "defensively closed type," a "carrier of a bodily veto" — is great and constant. This must not be done. A configuration in DDSRF is a map of the current assembly of experience, not a property of the person. The same client in whom a shame organization dominates today may come in tomorrow with an active grief organization, and a week later with a dissociative one. Configurations are not treated. They are read.

Diagnostic systems do other work — they categorize pathology, direct psychiatric treatment, ensure communication between clinicians. DDSRF does not replace any of these functions. The clinical category "depressive episode" and the assembly category "grief configuration with the veto on the side of narrative" are not synonyms. They are not even on the same axis. The first answers the question "what to prescribe and what to build a course of treatment around." The second — "what, at this moment of the session, holds the veto on the next step." Both can be used at once, and that is no contradiction. A contradiction arises only when the assembly language begins to claim to be diagnostic.

DDSRF is not a school of therapy. It has no techniques of its own. All techniques remain with the schools the therapist draws them from. If someone says, "I work in the DDSRF approach," this is already a distortion. A therapist may work in a psychoanalytic, CBT, ACT, Gestalt, EMDR, body-oriented, or existential approach and read the moment through DDSRF. This does not make DDSRF an approach. It makes it a grammar on which different approaches can speak.

The distinction matters. An approach gives the therapist what to do. A grammar gives them how to read the moment in which they do something. These two functions are not interchangeable. A therapist without an approach is at a loss. A therapist without a grammar is precise, but sometimes prematurely right. The book works at the second level and makes no claim on the first.

DDSRF does not solve the problem of consciousness. The two-domain structure we will unfold in Chapter 3 is a methodological discipline, not an ontological solution. DDSRF does not explain why subjective experience exists, how experience arises from neural activity, or what the nature of the relation between the P-domain and the M-domain is. These questions remain open, and DDSRF does not close them. It works at a level below the philosophy of consciousness and above neurobiology — at the level of clinical methodology.

This must be said plainly, because theories that hold phenomenology and mechanism together at once tend to slide either into reduction (everything is explicable by mechanics) or into emergentist rhetoric (experience is irreducible, full stop). DDSRF does neither. It requires clinicians to hold both domains as mutual constraints and does not answer the question of exactly how they are connected. This is an honest "I don't know" at the foundation of the theory, not its weakness.

DDSRF is not a normative system of what should be integrated. Integrability is a descriptive construct. What exactly to integrate in each particular case is decided by the therapist together with the client, within their contract, ethics, and cultural context. DDSRF does not sanction "accepting the trauma," "working with shame," "opening up the future," or any other substantive goal as universally right. It shows only what can, right now, be integrated without overloading the system — and leaves the question "what to choose to integrate" entirely outside its competence.

This is especially important to say, because the very word "integration" in the clinical literature often carries a normative load — as if an integrated state were always better than a non-integrated one. In DDSRF this is not so. Sometimes the clinically right thing is not to integrate. Integration may mean a boundary, a refusal, a departure, anger, mourning, action, or a change of conditions — and this too widens subjective reality rather than narrowing it. More on this in §4.6, where integrability is unfolded as a clinical category. DDSRF is not a theory of obedience and not a theory of adaptation. It is a theory of how the new becomes part of lived reality — whatever that new may be.

DDSRF does not work with severe clinical conditions as a treatment protocol. Psychotic disorders, severe affective episodes, suicidal risk, eating disorders with medical decompensation, bipolar episodes, severe dissociative states — these are an area where the first work is done by psychiatry and specialized clinical training. DDSRF can read these states through its axes — for example, through the organization axis O1–O5, from stable assembly to psychotically disorganizing — but does not offer to treat them.

This is an honest boundary, and it must not be violated. The book is written for the practice in which most situations lie between these extremes: clients with a history of trauma, with moderate personality disorders, with depressive and anxious states, with existential crises, with difficulties of relationship and identity. In this zone DDSRF works. Beyond it, it remains readable as a language of description, but not as a guide to action.

2.4. Compatibility with schools as a practical test

There is a simple criterion by which to check whether DDSRF is being used correctly. If, after encountering the theory, a clinician has come to understand more precisely when their own method lands and when it is premature — DDSRF is working as intended. If they have abandoned their school for the sake of DDSRF — DDSRF has been used against its own nature.

The psychoanalyst remains a psychoanalyst after the reading. But sees more precisely: when an interpretation enters an open Cα mode and when it meets defensive closure; which layer assembles the current assembly and where the client holds a veto; what "the interpretation is premature here" means not in a general analytic sense but in an operational one.

The CBT therapist remains a CBT therapist. But sees more precisely: when a behavioral experiment rests on a sufficient reality weight of the alternative perspective, and when it runs into an RW4 configuration in which refutation does not land; when low "motivation" is a sign of unreadiness for this load right now, not a defect of the client.

The ACT practitioner remains an ACT practitioner. But sees more precisely: which layer of the system is, at this moment, sustaining "fusion," and what work with that layer will make cognitive defusion (defusion) possible; how pseudo-acceptance differs from the integrated kind.

The trauma therapist remains a trauma therapist. But gains a language in which the window of tolerance (window of tolerance), phase-based work, and titration cease to be trauma-therapy notions only, and become special cases of a more general fit between load and capacity. This gives them the ability to discuss their work with colleagues from other schools without translating through intuition.

The Gestalt therapist remains a Gestalt therapist. But gains an additional reading of what their language calls "interruption of contact": which interruption is a defensive closure after premature contact, and which is a stabilization before a step being prepared. A distinction that is hard to make cleanly within the Gestalt apparatus itself.

This list can be continued for DBT, EMDR, existential, body-oriented, systemic, and narrative approaches. The logic is the same in each case: DDSRF does not replace a school's language. It adds to it a layer for reading the moment, on which the languages of the schools begin to hear one another.

The reverse follows too. If a clinician, having taken up DDSRF, begins to devalue the schools — that is a sign the theory is being used against its purpose. DDSRF is not above psychoanalysis, not above CBT, not above

ACT. It is on a different plane. Arrogance in this direction is the most frequent form of its distortion, and it is worth naming directly.

2.5. What we now have and what comes next

The boundary of the theory is set. DDSRF has a subject (the clinical moment, read as a fit between load and capacity), a method (two-domain reading of the assembly), working categories (which we will unfold in the following chapters), and honest “no”s in the places where the theory does not work.

Next we must begin the language itself. The central category, without which none of the later concepts has support, is subjective reality. This is the working name for what is, at a given moment, assembled in the client as the lived. Not an image of the world. Not a schema. Not beliefs. What is, for them, real right now. With all the force that distinguishes the real from the understood, the considered, or the imagined.

And in parallel — the two-domain structure as a methodological discipline that keeps the theory from two typical slides: into pure phenomenology without conditions, and into pure mechanism without experience.

These two themes — subjective reality and the two-domain architecture — are the subject of Chapter 3.

Chapter 3. Subjective Reality and the Two-Domain Architecture

3.1. What exactly is assembled

A single phrase has run through the book from the start, one we have not yet fully unpacked: the client's subjective reality cannot integrate this right now. We spoke of premature rightness as an action right in content that does not land. We said that the client's system protects its integrity. But what is this system? What exactly is it that "cannot integrate" — and what is it made of?

Take a scene. A man around forty comes in and says: "I haven't felt anything for my wife for months. I don't know if I love her. I'm thinking about divorce." One therapist will hear here a loss of meaning, an existential crisis, perhaps the echo of an early loss — and will follow the line of experience. Another will hear anhedonia, possible depression, exhaustion, a hormonal background — and will follow the line of conditions. Both may be right. But if it turns out that the client began taking a medication six months ago and the emotional flattening appeared around the same time, the order of work changes. This does not cancel the existential material. But first — a conversation about the medication, and then whatever remains once that condition is taken into account.

This scene shows two things at once. First: the client's experience has a form — how exactly the absence of feeling is experienced, whether it is emptiness, frozenness, or distance — and it has conditions without which that form does not change. Second: what the client brings as a single "I don't feel anything" is in fact assembled out of many things — out of the body, out of the medication's chemistry, out of the history of the marriage, out of how he has grown used to experiencing closeness. This chapter is about how the system that assembles lived reality is built, and why working with it requires two different languages of description. Everything to be built in the following chapters — fit, Cα modes, reality weight, the dominant constraint, sequence, the counter-experience — will rest on this architecture. Here we describe it.

3.2. Subjective reality is assembled, not reflected

DDSRF calls the client's actual lived reality R(t) — the configuration of world, self, other, time, body, and action as it is for the person at a given moment. It is worth saying at once what R(t) is not. It is not a picture of the world, not beliefs, not a schema, not the story the client tells about themselves. It is what is real for them right now — with the force that distinguishes the real from the understood, the considered, or the imagined. A client may understand that they are not being rejected and still live in the reality of rejection. R(t) is the second one — the one that weighs as world.

And the key point: R(t) is assembled. It does not reflect an external state of affairs, does not receive it passively, does not interpret ready-made material — it assembles the lived whole anew, at every moment. Subjective reality is not a receiver that takes in information and stores it. It is an active organization that at every moment decides — not consciously, but at the level of assembly — what will enter, what will bounce off, what will turn into confirmation of the already known, and what will trigger collapse. When later in the book we say that an intervention "does not land," we are describing precisely this decision of the assembly. It is not made by the client deliberately and is not the therapist's fault. It is the work of a system that assembles reality and protects its coherence.

From this it is clear why "explaining to the client how things really are" so often does not work. The explanation is addressed to the picture of the world — but suffering is governed not by the picture but by the assembled reality. For something to change, that reality must be reassembled, not the map refined.

3.3. Cα and the layers of assembly

If R(t) is assembled, we need a way to describe the operation of assembly itself. DDSRF calls this operation Cα — the assembly operator: that which binds the inputs from several layers into a single lived whole. A caveat at once, to avoid misunderstanding: Cα is not a proven mechanism and not a hidden organ of the psyche. It is a conceptual name for an operation we observe through its result — through disparate layers becoming one lived reality.

There are seven layers from which the assembly draws: predictive activity and its precision (Pσ), the intersubjective field of the other (S(t)), the narrative layer of meanings and stories (N(t)), the bodily base and autonomic regulation (B(t)), the thresholds of coherence and transformation (Θ), the developmental calibration of early experience (D_cal), and the context of the life-world (Λ). Each of these layers will later become a working instrument: it is among them that Chapter 7 will look for the one holding the veto. What matters here is something else — not what each layer does separately, but that Cα does not sum them, it binds them.

In working notation this can be written:

R(t) = Cα [Pσ, S(t), N(t), B(t), Θ, D_cal, Λ]

This notation is not a mathematical equation. It computes nothing and predicts no outcome. It only holds in one line what the clinician must not lose: subjective reality is assembled through several layers at once, not from a single source.

This distinction matters. The body of a client experiencing threat does not exist apart from their prediction of threat, from the field of the other who may hold or amplify it, from the story in which the threat took shape, from the early calibration that makes it recognizable, and from the context that confirms or refutes it. All of this is assembled into one — into the lived reality of threat, where the layers are no longer separable from one another. This is why a single layer may be an entry point but is rarely a full explanation: the other layers hold the assembly and often return it to its prior state. And this is why, in Chapter 7, we will look not for "the main layer in general" but for the layer that right now holds the veto on the next step.

3.4. Why suffering is stable: assembly is recursive

The assembly has a property that explains why subjective reality is so hard to change. It is recursive: what is assembled as R(t) now becomes a condition of the assembly of R(t+1) at the next moment.

Look at how this works. A client experiences the other as dangerous — and closes down. The other, in response, reacts more coldly. The coldness confirms the prediction of danger. The body strengthens its defense. The narrative "people cannot be trusted" grows firmer. The thresholds of coherence drop. And the next encounter is assembled as a threat — already stronger than before. No one designed this cycle; it assembles itself. Each turn makes the old reality a little more real.

This is the self-reproducing loop of subjective reality, and it is what makes suffering stable. Here it is worth clarifying a word that will recur in the book: configuration. A configuration is not just a recurring pattern of experience. It is a pattern that confirms itself in each subsequent cycle of assembly. The difference is decisive for the work: a recurring pattern can be interrupted by pointing it out; a self-confirming configuration cannot be interrupted by pointing, because it will build the very pointing into its cycle. This is why change requires not only a new understanding but a new experience (Chapter 9): a lived event that the old configuration cannot immediately turn into its own confirmation — and so, for the first time, it makes the loop not the only one.

3.5. The therapist assembles reality together with the client

From the fact that one of the layers of the assembly is the field of the other, S(t), follows a conclusion easy to miss but that changes everything.

The therapist does not observe the client's R(t) from outside. The therapist is part of S(t). In the consulting room the client's reality is assembled not in front of the therapist but together with them. The therapist's voice, pace, pause, the capacity to bear the client's shame and not turn away, the readiness to stay in contact when the client expects rejection — all of this enters the assembly, becomes one of its layers here and now.

This has two consequences. First: S(t) is a layer in which the therapist participates not only through words but through the very manner of their presence. They cannot directly retune the client's body, their early calibration, or their life context — but they themselves, through their presence, are one of the layers from which the client's reality is assembled at this moment;

this is their most immediate point of participation in the assembly. The second consequence is what the book will later call dyadicity and counter-load. If the therapist cannot bear what rises in them — shame, helplessness, the urge to rescue or explain — the field breaks from their side, and the assembly registers it. The therapist's counter-load is not a sentimental addition to the "real" technical work. It is a structural part of how the client's reality is assembled.

3.6. Two languages of description: P and M

Now to what the whole chapter is for. The assembly has two sides, and each requires its own language. DDSRF calls them the P-domain and the M-domain and holds both — not as a philosophical compromise but as a working discipline.

The P-domain is the area of lived experience from within. Shame as the experience of a visibility that destroys. Anxiety as a real premonition of catastrophe, not as a "cognitive distortion." Time as a space expanding in hope and contracting in hopelessness. This is what the client comes with: they come not with a "malfunction of the serotonin system" but with the experience that the world has gone flat or that they are about to be judged. This experience has a form, a force, and an organization — and it is precisely this form that is the clinical material. The clinical entry most often begins with the P-domain, because the client brings experience; but the work must not stop there — any serious description of the form requires the question of the conditions that sustain it.

The M-domain is the mechanistic domain, or, more broadly, the domain of conditions that sustain this experience while not themselves being it. The word "mechanistic" here does not mean only the brain or biology: it means everything that sustains, constrains, or makes possible a given form of experience while not being that form. The body and the autonomic regulation without which coherence falls apart. Sleep, in the lack of which predictions become unsteady and threat is read where there is none. The hormonal background, the action of medications, hypoglycemia. Attachment patterns as early predictions of how the other will behave. And — no less — the external context: family, work, economic and legal standing, environment. A person experiencing the world as dangerous may live in a genuinely dangerous environment, and this is part of the M-domain no less than the workings of their autonomic system. The M-domain is not reducible to the brain: it is conditions in general — bodily, behavioral, relational, environmental.

Why both. Experience does not hang in the air — it has conditions, and to ignore them is to conduct therapy in a vacuum. But the conditions are not the experience itself, and to reduce experience to them is to lose the very thing the person came for. The two-domain discipline requires holding both registers at once: while listening to the client, reading the form of their experience and seeing the conditions in which that form became possible. Not in turn — first phenomenology, then mechanism — but as two layers of one reading. This is harder than working in one language, and so it is not the most habitual skill. Most of us slip more quickly into one register — the phenomenological or the mechanistic.

3.7. What the two-domain structure is not

Three denials are important to state plainly, because without them the two-domain structure is easily taken for what it is not.

It is not dualism. DDSRF does not claim that there are two separate substances — experience and matter — that interact mysteriously. The distinction between P and M is methodological, not ontological: these are two levels of description of one and the same event, not two different worlds. When a client experiences shame, that is one event. From the P-side it is described as the experience of a destroying visibility, with all its form and history. From the M-side — as a state of the body, a configuration of predictions, a context of relationships. One event, two languages. The error begins where one language declares itself the only one.

It is not reductionism. DDSRF does not say that experience "really is" mechanism — that shame "is" a pattern of activation, that anxiety "is" a state of the autonomic system. This is a category error, and it is clinically dangerous: if shame is a pattern, then working with shame reduces to changing the pattern, and the form of the experience — its content, history, organization — disappears. Symmetrically, DDSRF does not reduce the conditions to experience either: an exhausted body, a dangerous environment, hypoglycemia are real in themselves. The two-domain discipline refuses both reductions.

It is not a solution to the hard problem of consciousness (hard problem). Why subjective experience exists at all, why the processing of information is accompanied by experience from within — this question DDSRF does not touch. It works one level below: not "why is there experience" but "how is the experience that already exists organized"; not "how does experience arise" but "why does this experience carry such weight that it governs a life despite rational disagreement." The nature of the connection between P and M remains an open philosophical question, and DDSRF says honestly that it does not solve it. This is a deliberate self-limitation: a clinical theory that claims to solve the hard problem of consciousness either overrates itself or substitutes therapy for philosophy.

3.8. Two symmetrical errors

The practical value of the two-domain structure is that it protects against two errors into which both beginning and experienced clinicians fall. It matters that they are symmetrical: neither the biological nor the phenomenological tilt is safer than the other.

P-reduction — more precisely, reducing the clinical reading to the P-domain alone — is working only with experience while ignoring the conditions. A client speaks of chronic fatigue, loss of interest, slowed thinking; the therapist works with this as an existential crisis or a depressive defense — and the client has untreated hypothyroidism, and until the thyroid is corrected, work with meaning will yield no result. P-reduction forgets that experience has a body, and the body has a vote. The same goes for working with a traumatic intrusion as "material to be worked through" when the threshold of coherence is too low and the working-through fragments; or working with a person in a genuinely dangerous environment as though their sense of danger were a distorted perception.

M-reduction — reducing the clinical reading to conditions and mechanisms — is explaining experience by mechanism so confidently that the experience itself ceases to be the object of the work. A client experiences shame; the therapist replies: "this is activation of the social-threat system, the amygdala is over-reacting." The explanation may be correct — and at the same time it closes the work: the client receives a frame in which their shame is not their experience but a biological process, and the form of the experience disappears. The same goes for turning polyvagal theory or predictive processing into ready answers instead of clinical material; for the conviction that stabilizing the autonomic system is therapy, rather than its condition.

And an important caveat about tone, because this chapter reads easily as an argument with biology. It is not an argument. The M-domain is real and sometimes clinically decisive: sometimes the first thing to do is to fix sleep, adjust a medication, assess the thyroid, help someone leave a dangerous environment. Biological and mechanistic models are neither naive nor hostile — they describe real conditions. The error is not in using them, but in replacing one side of the description with the other. The two-domain discipline keeps the therapist from both reductions by requiring, at every moment, the question: what am I reading right now — the form of the experience or its conditions? And am I missing the other?

3.9. What the method will stand on

The architecture is in place. We have described what DDSRF calls subjective reality R(t), why it is assembled through Cα, why the assembly is multilayered, why suffering reproduces itself, why the therapist enters S(t), and why clinical work needs two languages of description — the form of experience and its conditions.

From here the book will unfold this architecture into a method, and each subsequent concept will describe something within it. Clinical integrability (Chapter 4) is the question of what the assembly of R(t) is currently able to take in. Cα modes (Chapter 5) are states of the assembly operator itself. Reality weight (Chapter 6) is the force with which the assembled reality acts as the only one possible. The dominant constraint (Chapter 7) is the search for the layer of the assembly that currently holds the veto. The principle of sequence (Chapter 8) is the grammar of the order in which the assembly is able to reassemble. The counter-experience (Chapter 9) is the small lived thing that the recursive loop does not manage to absorb, and which therefore begins to change it.

It begins with one question. If R(t) is assembled and protects its coherence, then not every intervention, even one right in content, can enter it. We need to understand when new material becomes fit for the current assembly. This is the question of clinical integrability — and it is where DDSRF's reading of the moment begins.

Part II

Reading the Clinical Moment

Chapter 4. Clinical Integrability

4.1. Two sessions with the same client

A client of forty-five, a history of marked paternal dysfunction, a long-standing pattern of self-criticism that he already understands well. Therapeutic work in its third year. The alliance is strong, the reflective capacity high.

A session in April. The client brings, for the first time, a dream in which he refuses to embrace his father. His voice trembles. The therapist says — calmly, in the right pause: "It seems you've let yourself, for the first time, not want to come close to him." The client nods. He is silent for a few seconds. His breathing evens out. He says: "Yes. It's a strange feeling." For the next ten minutes both stay with this. At the end of the session the client says he feels lighter. The following week he reports that after the session, for the first time in years, he was able to say "no" to his partner in a situation where he would previously have agreed automatically.

A session in October, six months later. The same client, the same theme — the relationship with the father. But two details set this session apart from April's. At the start the client mentions in passing that he does not want to turn therapy back into "talk about childhood" — he came to discuss the present. And two exchanges later it emerges that a week ago the father called again and spoke to him in that same old, humiliating tone. The therapist says, in the same intonation as in April: "It seems you don't want to come close to him now either." The client falls silent. His face hardens. He says in a level voice: "Maybe. I don't know. It's probably infantile." The rest of the session passes formally. A week later the client comes in and reports that he has thought a great deal and decided to "work more constructively, without this childish acting-out."

The same intervention. The same client. The same therapist. A different result.

The difference can be read. In April the intervention entered what we will later call a transitional mode of assembly: the client could experience "I may not come close" as a new possibility. In October the same sentence landed in a different assembly. The day before, the old paternal calibration had been reactivated — a call in a humiliating tone returned the client to the position of "the small one." And he himself came already fearing that the work would again turn into a "childish" conversation about the past. So the intervention was heard not as permission for a boundary but as a threat of regression: "I'm infantile again, I haven't grown up after all." The content of the intervention barely changed. The mode of assembly changed. And so its fit changed.

If one tries to explain this difference through the content of the intervention, nothing comes of it: the content matches almost word for word. Through the client — he is the same, and in theory has become more "integrated" over six months, not less. Through the alliance — it was not harmed. Through readiness — on the surface the client came in October more composed than in April. None of the usual categories explains the difference.

DDSRF offers a category that does explain it. It is clinical integrability: in April the client's system could take in this intervention without closing down; in October it could not. Not because the client got worse. But because in October the assembly of the moment was different — a different current capacity, a different load of the same intervention, a different state of the field. The difference between these two sessions is the subject of this whole chapter.

4.2. What integrative capacity is

Integrative capacity is the ability of the client's current assembly to hold, process, and take in new material without losing coherence and without closing down. Not the potential ability. Not the ability "in general." The current one — now, at this moment, with this assembly, this body, this field, this history behind it. One can picture it as the system's throughput for the new — but this metaphor is useful only until it starts to sound like something measurable in units. Capacity is not measured. It is read.

It is worth saying at once what integrative capacity is not. This will help see more precisely what it is.

It is not readiness for change. Readiness says whether the client wants to. Capacity says whether the current system can take in the new — regardless of whether the client wants to or not. One can passionately want to change with low capacity. One can want nothing with high capacity — no one has yet made use of it.

It is not level of functioning. Functioning says how a person holds life as a whole. Capacity says whether they can take in precisely this material precisely now. A high-functioning client with a mobilized defensive assembly may have less capacity for a given intervention than a less functional one whose defense is not currently raised.

It is not the alliance. The alliance says whether there is a connection and of what quality. Capacity says what, within that connection, the system is able to process. A good alliance can coexist with low capacity for a specific intervention — for example, when the client deeply trusts the therapist but, for that very reason, is not now ready to hear it said aloud. The alliance protects against closing-down after a premature intervention, but does not cancel its prematureness.

It is not ego strength, not personality structure, not frustration tolerance. All these constructs concern long-term characteristics. Integrative capacity concerns the local state of the assembly now. The same client with the same ego strength has, at different moments of the day, different capacity for one and the same intervention. In the morning after a bad night's sleep — one. After a calm weekend — another. After a hard conversation on the way to the session — a third. This does not mean capacity is a capricious, unstable thing that cannot be relied on. It means it is read in the moment, not assumed from history.

And, finally, something important. Integrative capacity is not a moral characteristic. Low capacity does not mean the client is "weak," "immature," or "resisting." It is a local state of the system that has its own causes — bodily, narrative, contextual, developmental. A therapist who assesses capacity is not assessing the client. They are reading what is possible now.

If capacity exists and is read, a new clinical question appears: what currently determines it? And this question leads us straight to the notion of the dominant constraint in Chapter 7. One of the system's layers — the body, the field of the other, narrative, predictive activity, developmental calibration, the context of the life-world — has, at each moment, the greatest influence on capacity, and sometimes a veto. To find this layer is the central methodological task of reading the moment.

For now this is enough. We have a working name for one side of clinical integrability. We need the second.

4.3. The load of the intervention

The load of the intervention is the demand the intervention places on the client's system in order to be integrated. Not the complexity of the intervention. Not its rightness. Not its affective intensity. Precisely — how much integration work it requires.

The load has at least three sides important for clinical reading. The first is the content side. What exactly the intervention proposes to integrate. A new formulation of a feeling ("this seems to be not anger but shame"), for instance, is one load. A new formulation of the relationship with a significant figure ("your mother in this story was not a protector but a source of danger") is another, usually considerably higher. A behavioral experiment with a situation the client has avoided for years is a third. Content load differs by which layers of the assembly it touches and how deeply it intrudes into the current R(t).

The second side is the manner of introduction. The same content load, delivered differently, can become a different load. An interpretation voiced as the therapist's assertion loads more heavily than the same interpretation offered as a hypothesis. The client's affect named and addressed directly to them loads more heavily than the same affect indicated obliquely. A named significant figure — father, mother, former partner — loads more heavily than the abstract figure of "a significant other." Each of these differences is not stylistic. It is a different load on the same assembly.

The third side, and often the decisive one, is which old reality the intervention contradicts. The same sentence carries a different load for different clients depending on how far it collides with what is, for them, real right now. "You may disagree" is almost zero load for a client to whom disagreement is already available. And very high — for one whose entire subjective reality has for years rested on the prohibition of disagreement: for them this sentence is not information but an assault on the structure of the world. The load, then, is not a property of the intervention in itself. It arises at the meeting of the intervention with a specific current assembly. How to read the force of that meeting we will return to when we speak of the reality weight of experience (Chapter 6) and of which layer of the system holds the assembly (Chapter 7).

All three sides act together. High-load content, delivered as a careful hypothesis in the right moment of pause and not colliding head-on with the client's old reality, may turn out to be integrable. The same content, voiced as a confident interpretation in a moment of the client's mobilization, may not land. And symmetrically: low-load content, delivered at the wrong moment or with the wrong density, may also fail to land. This is what it means that an action right in content is not identical to a fit action — what was named in Chapter 1 as premature rightness.

Here a caveat important for practice. Load is not equal to intensity. A quiet sentence said at the right moment may carry a higher load than a dramatic interpretation. And conversely: an outwardly "strong" intervention may carry minimal load if it simply names what the client has almost said themselves. A therapist who orients to intensity systematically misses the load. A therapist who orients to load sometimes says the quietest sentences at the most pivotal moments — and they land.

4.4. The formula that holds the whole book

We have two sides. On one — the current integrative capacity of the system. On the other — the load of the intervention. Between them — a relation that determines what becomes possible.

An intervention becomes clinically fit when its load falls into the zone of fit with integrative capacity. If such a fit intervention creates a minimal counter-experience, change can begin.

It is worth saying at once why the formula is stated this way — through fit and possibility, not through "change happens." A fit between load and capacity does not guarantee change. It makes change possible. For change to actually occur, more is needed: a counter-experience, its holding, its repeatability, its integration through body, relationship, narrative, and action. That is the subject of Chapter 9. The formula of fit is a necessary condition, not a sufficient one. This distinction matters to keep, otherwise the theory begins to sound as if a correctly dosed intervention by itself produces change. It only opens the way to it.

Next, what the formula asserts and what it does not.

It asserts: the fit is two-sided. An excess of load over capacity yields premature rightness: an intervention right in content does not land, because the system cannot hold it. An excess of capacity over load yields perpetual stabilization: capacity is there, the new is available — but no intervention brings into the system a load sufficient for a counter-experience. Both situations are clinically real and both are called errors in DDSRF (Chapter 1).

It asserts: the fit is not a point-equality but a working zone. An intervention is fit not when it is "perfectly dosed" but when its load is in the working zone: large enough to create the possibility of the new, and small enough not to cause closing-down or collapse. DDSRF is not a theory of dosage. It is a theory of reading the zone of fit. In the trauma-therapy tradition, the metaphor of the window of tolerance is used for a closely related notion. DDSRF accepts this intuition and generalizes it: the window of tolerance is a special case of the zone of fit, localized in bodily-affective regulation. The zone of fit spans all layers of the assembly, not only the bodily one.

It does not assert: that the fit is about caution. DDSRF is not a theory of "do not load the client." Sometimes the fit requires increasing the load — because without it the client stays in a zone where the new is impossible. Sometimes the fit requires decreasing it. Sometimes the fit requires silence. The decision depends not on a theoretical preference for one side but on what the reading of current capacity and current load shows.

And — most important — the formula does not assert that the fit concerns the client only. That is the next step.

4.5. Why integrability is dyadic

In the previous section the formula was stated deliberately incompletely. The full formulation reads:

An intervention becomes clinically fit when its load falls into the zone of fit with the integrative capacity of the client, the therapist, and the field between them.

This is not a sentimental extension. It is a structural assertion, and it changes the whole practice of reading the moment.

The client has a capacity for a given intervention. The therapist has one too. Put this way the thought is less familiar, but on inspection it is obvious. A therapist who voices an interpretation must be able to hold it after voicing: to hold the client's silence, their closing-down, possible anger, a possible "you understand nothing," a possible silent turning-away at the next session. If the therapist cannot hold this counter-load, they either withdraw the interpretation (through softening, qualification, premature reassurance), or double it (through insistence, the wish to convince, elaboration), or begin to apologize. Each of these movements breaks the field, and the intervention, however right in content, ceases to be fit.

The therapist's capacity is their ability to hold their own counter-load: shame at their own possible error, helplessness, the urge to rescue, fear of losing the client, fear of their own envy, fear of their own emptiness. Each of these internal loads can overload the therapist at a moment still passable for the client. And then the client remains all right, while what breaks is the field — from the therapist's side.

The clinical tradition has long known this problem — through the language of countertransference, of bearing, of presence, and of supervisory work. DDSRF formulates it differently: as the counter-load of the intervention. This is not a new theme, but a new way of including it in the assessment of an action's fit. An intervention may be non-integrable not only because the client cannot withstand it, but because the therapist or the field cannot withstand the consequences of introducing it. Thereby the therapist's counter-load becomes symmetrical to the client's load — a part of the clinical methodology itself, not a supervisory addition to it.

From this follows a practical conclusion. Before every loading intervention the therapist must read not only the client but also themselves. This is not affective slowing and not self-rumination. It is a direct methodological question: "If this intervention causes closing-down, anger, or denial, will I be able to stay with it, without withdrawing it, without doubling it, and without apologizing?" If the answer is "no," the intervention is not fit, however right in content it may be. Not because the client cannot withstand it. Because the therapist cannot.

And there is a third element — the field S(t), the space of meeting itself. It too has a capacity, and it is often missed. The field may be thin — after a break, after a difficult previous session, at the start of the work, in the moment after a crisis. The field may be dense — after long shared work, after a crisis the pair lived through together. The same intervention in a thin field and in a dense field is a different load. And sometimes the work consists not in choosing the right intervention but in waiting until the field is dense enough to withstand it.

The full dyadic formula reads: an intervention is fit if all three — client, therapist, and field — can hold its load. If even one of the three cannot, the intervention loses its fit, regardless of what happens with the other two. This gives three places to check before every loading intervention, not one.

4.6. A descriptive, not a normative construct

It must be repeated — because everything depends on it — what was already said in Chapter 2. Clinical integrability is a descriptive construct, not a normative one.

DDSRF does not say what should be integrated. It says what can be integrated now. What to choose for integration is decided by the therapist together with the client, within their contract, ethics, and cultural context.

This is important to say, because the very word "integration" in the clinical literature often carries the load of "integrated is better than non-integrated." In DDSRF this is not so. Sometimes the clinically correct thing is not to integrate. Sometimes the right integration is the integration of separation, refusal, anger, mourning, departure. A client may integrate "that was abuse," "I am no longer obliged to endure this," "this environment is destroying me," "I am leaving this." That is full integration, and it widens the client's subjective reality rather than narrowing it.

From this follows one thing worth naming directly. The therapist errs not when they take integrability into account in choosing an intervention — that is exactly what is necessary. The error begins where integrability becomes the only criterion for choosing the content of the work. “This is integrable now — so this is what should be introduced” is a misuse of the theory. Integrability answers the question “can this land now.” It does not answer the question “is this clinically, ethically, and contractually important.” The second question is decided within the therapeutic contract, the method, ethics, culture, and the client’s concrete situation — and DDSRF does not answer it.

And symmetrically: a therapist who uses low integrability as a justification for not bringing something essential into the work also errs. “This is non-integrable now, so I will not” is sometimes the right clinical decision and sometimes a form of perpetual stabilization. The two can be told apart only through reading what happens over time: if capacity for this material does not grow over time, because the therapist never takes steps toward it, this is no longer respect for the client but avoidance of one’s own counter-load.

4.7. A first map of integrability

So far the chapter has explained integrability. Now — a first way to read it. Before a significant intervention, the therapist can ask themselves six questions.

1. **What exactly am I about to introduce?** Not “what do I want to say,” but what new material, experience, or distinction am I offering the client’s system.
2. **What load does this create for the client?** What will the client have to withstand if the intervention lands: shame, anger, a new view of the other, the giving-up of an old narrative, bodily activation, the risk of action?
3. **What is the client’s integrative capacity right now?** Can the current assembly hold this material without closing down, without falling apart, and without turning it into pseudo-agreement?
4. **What will this intervention require of me as the therapist?** Will I be able to withstand silence, anger, denial, shame, dependency, devaluation, or my own urge to soften what was said?
5. **What can the field between us withstand right now?** Is the field S(t) currently dense enough that the intervention will not be heard as intrusion, judgment, pressure, or withdrawal?

6. **If this is premature, what must become possible first?** What smaller step will increase capacity: body, field, language, pace, safety, distinction, context?

This is not a checklist for mechanical application. It is a way to stop premature rightness before it happens. The full version of this map is given in the DDSRF Case Card in the Method Atlas (Appendix A). What matters here is not the form but the logic itself: an intervention is assessed not only by its content but by its fit — for the client, the therapist, and the field.

4.8. What to measure and what not to measure

There is sometimes a temptation to turn integrability into a quantitative scale — to give the client a "capacity score," give the intervention a "load score," subtract one from the other, and obtain a ready decision. This should not be done.

Not because measurement is bad in principle. But because local measurement in the clinical moment usually creates false precision. The clinician has instruments that help read the state of the assembly qualitatively — Cα modes (Chapter 5), the reality weight of experience (Chapter 6), the dominant constraint (Chapter 7). These instruments give distinctions, not numbers. The distinction between a defensively closed and a stabilizing mode, between RW2 and RW4, between a bodily and a narrative veto — that is what changes a clinical decision. No integral figure of "capacity 6.2 / load 7.1" gives anything beyond these distinctions, and usually it takes the living reading away from the clinician.

Nonetheless, the Method Atlas contains a working instrument — the Load–Capacity–Field Grid (Appendix E) — which structures the reading of load and capacity along three axes (client, therapist, field) and helps notice an imbalance that might otherwise be missed. It is not a scale and not a calculator. It is a map that makes the dyadic reading explicit. For those who want a reference instrument at hand, it is there. For those for whom a qualitative reading is enough, the main text of the book gives everything needed.

One sentence is worth remembering, because it holds the entire epistemic discipline of this chapter. DDSRF does not measure integrability. DDSRF distinguishes the signs of integrability. A distinction — not a number — is what changes a clinical decision.

4.9. Where we go next

We now have three working notions — integrative capacity, the load of the intervention, the dyadic completeness of their fit — and a first map of six questions that translates them into practice. Two of those questions the map already poses, but does not yet itself supply criteria for answering. "What is the client's capacity right now?" and "what can the field withstand?" are questions about the state of the assembly in the moment, and to answer them precisely, rather than by eye, one needs reading instruments. There are three, and each answers its own sub-question.

In which mode of assembly is the client working right now? — this is answered by the Cα mode map (Chapter 5). The five modes — fragmenting, defensively closed, stabilizing, exploratory, transitional — are distinguished not by the content of experience but by what the system does with novelty.

With what reality weight of experience are we working? — this is answered by the reality weight scale RW0–RW4 (Chapter 6). From semantic content that does not govern, to a self-enclosed reality into which refutation barely enters.

Which layer of the system currently holds the veto on the next step? — this is answered by the dominant constraint protocol (Chapter 7). Seven layers of assembly, three statuses for each, three tests for determining the veto, the rule of triangulation.

Each of these three chapters is a next step in building the instrument that will allow the moment to be read precisely enough to turn the formula of fit into a working category of clinical practice.

We begin with the Cα modes — because they give the first, largest distinction on which the others rest.

Chapter 5. Cα Modes

5.1. One session, four modes

The client sits across and talks about a quarrel with his brother. He speaks coherently, ironically, even with interest in his own reaction: “Funny, I’ve turned into a resentful teenager again.” This is already a view of himself from outside — he is examining his reaction, not only living in it.

The therapist gently suggests looking at what exactly in the brother he reacts to so sharply. And the client suddenly changes. His voice becomes level and quick: “Well yes, my brother was always the favorite, there’s nothing to explore here, it’s just a fact.” The curiosity is gone. Any attempt to look differently now bounces off — turns into confirmation of what is already known.

The therapist notices this and does not press. He speaks more quietly, offers no versions, simply stays alongside and observes: “It seems this is hard to talk about other than the way you’re used to.” The client is silent. Then, more slowly: “Yes. I don’t know how else. But I hear that you’re not arguing.” The voice lets go a little. He is not yet open, but no longer sealed shut.

And a few minutes later, when the therapist asks what is hardest in this role of “the unloved one,” the client answers, for the first time, not from a position but from experience. His eyes fill. “What’s hard is that I still want it. At forty. From a person who doesn’t care.” His voice trembles, but he does not fall apart. Something new is said for the first time and is held.

In twenty minutes the client’s system passed through four different states. First it explored. Then it closed. Then it began to reassemble. Then, for a second, it let the new in and held it. The content all this time was one — the relationship with the brother. What changed was not the content. What changed was what the system, at each moment, did with the new.

The fifth mode — the fragmenting one — did not arise in this scene. And that matters: the work became possible precisely because, under strong affect at the end, coherence did not fall apart. Had it been weaker, that same moment could have turned not into a transition but into collapse.

This is the subject of the chapter. The assembly of subjective reality — Cα, the operator that binds all the layers into a single lived whole — has, at every moment, a mode. And the mode is determined not by what the client says but by what happens to novelty after its contact with the system.

It is worth saying at once what "novelty" means in this chapter. It is not only new information and not only a new thought of the therapist. Novelty can be an interpretation, a pause, a question, an emotion, a bodily sensation, a surfaced memory, a change in the therapist's tone, a small action of the client themselves, the appearance of another point of view — or the very fact that old, familiar material is, for the first time, experienced differently. Novelty is everything that requires the current subjective reality to update. This is why the mode is read through the handling of novelty: it is the most general test of what the system is currently able to do.

5.2. First, the main point: modes are not stages

Before listing the modes, we must say what, without which, the whole map will be misunderstood.

Cα modes are not stages of therapy and not phases of the client's development. They are states of the assembly at a given moment. The client does not "pass through" them once in the right order — from fragmentation to transition, as up a staircase. They move between them constantly, in both directions, sometimes within minutes, like the client in 5.1 who passed through four modes in twenty minutes. A mode is not what the client is. It is the state in which their assembly is working right now.

From this follows a practical conclusion. One cannot say "this client is in the exploratory mode" as a characteristic. One can say only "right now, at this moment, their assembly is working in the exploratory mode." Ten minutes later this may be untrue. The mode is read anew as often as what happens to novelty changes.

This distinction — between a mode as a state of the moment and a mode as a property of the person — is the same discipline we will hold in Chapter

7, when we turn to the dominant constraint: the instrument describes the current assembly, it does not make a diagnosis. The mode map is an instrument for the clinical reading of the moment; it helps read what is happening now, it does not classify the client.

5.3. The three axes through which a mode is read

A mode is not a label but a configuration of three assembly parameters. Each mode has its own profile of the three.

The first axis is **coherence**: is subjective reality held as a whole? Is experience not falling apart, is the thread holding, does the client remain in contact with body, time, place, therapist?

The second axis is **permeability**: can the system, right now, take in something new? Or does the new bounce off, fail to enter, turn into confirmation of the already known?

The third axis is **integrability**: can the new become part of experience, not only information? This is the highest bar — that very difference between "I heard it" and "it became part of how I experience myself," on which the whole book rests.

These three axes are not independent, but neither do they reduce to one another. One can have high coherence and almost absent permeability — this is closedness. One can have rising coherence and still-weak integrability — this is an assembly that is only just recovering. The five modes are five characteristic combinations of the three axes, and each calls for its own handling.

5.4. The five modes

The fragmenting mode. Novelty or the current material has exceeded coherence, and experience begins to fall apart. Speech loses the thread, breaks off, drifts into abstraction; panic, emptiness, derealization appear; contact with body, time, therapist is lost; what was just said is not held. Here neither interpretation nor deepening nor "stay with this experience" works, still less traumatic material or confrontation — all of this adds load where the system is already overwhelmed. Here the main work is one: to restore coherence.

Body, breath, orientation in the room, the therapist's voice, slowing the pace, calm presence. Until coherence is restored, no content work is fit.

The defensively closed mode. Coherence is preserved — the client speaks coherently, clearly, sometimes persuasively — but novelty is not let through. Any alternative turns into confirmation of the old reality ("that's exactly what I'm saying") or is devalued. Support is read as misunderstanding. And the main marker: after a good, accurate intervention there is more defense, not more space. This is the mode in which it is easiest to do harm, by taking the closedness for stubbornness and increasing the pressure. Arguing with the content, repeating the interpretation in other words, going "but" against the defense, trying to break through — all of this strengthens the closing. The reverse works: offer less, be present more, lower the threat of novelty, search through the field — through attunement, pace, pause — for what exactly this closing is defending.

The stabilizing mode. The system is still fragile, novelty is not yet integrated — but, unlike the closed mode, it is not rejected. Coherence is growing. The client may say "I can't go there yet," but not "this is useless." After regulation a little more contact appears. Material can be named without collapse. Here the work is to strengthen — body, field, the threshold of coherence — to name the state without interpretation, to hold the client's pace, to give space and not fill the pauses. Here the main work is to increase capacity, not to introduce new load before its time. And here is the main temptation, discussed in more detail below: not to mistake stabilization for therapy itself and not to get stuck in it forever.

The exploratory mode. Curiosity appears. The client says "maybe," "what if it's different," "I'm not sure"; is ready to consider other versions; is able to hold uncertainty and ambivalence; irony and humor without sarcasm are possible. Thought widens rather than narrows. Here distinction works — what is the same, what is genuinely different — along with alternative formulations, thought experiments, small trials; here the ground is prepared for a possible counter-experience. Two dangers. The first — to take intellectual agreement for integration: the client considers a new version with the mind, but this does not yet mean it has become part of their reality. The second — to remain in this mode for a long time without movement, and then therapy turns into a fine conversation in which everything is understood and nothing changes.

The transitional mode. The old and new realities coexist, and the new possibility ceases to be a thought — it begins to be experienced. The affect is strong, but coherence holds. A bodily trace of the new appears: the breathing changes, the posture lets go, it becomes possible to stay in contact. The client says "strange," "this is different," "I don't know what this is." The old is still present but no longer seizes the whole. The moment has a quality of aliveness. This is the mode in which a counter-experience can cease to be preparation or thought and begin to be experienced as reality (on which, Chapter 9), and it must be handled especially carefully. The worst thing one can do is to explain the moment, to close it with a quick generalization, to turn it into insight through "so, now you see that..." The experience makes itself; the therapist's task is to hold the moment, to name what is happening sparingly, to help the new take hold through body, relationship, narrative, and action, and not to forget that this mode is fragile and can roll back within minutes.

5.5. The distinction that decides the most: closed or stabilizing

Of the five modes, two are confused more often than all the rest combined — the defensively closed and the stabilizing. Outwardly they are alike: both can look calm, in both the client is not moving toward the new, in both coherence is preserved. And they are handled in exactly opposite ways. To confuse them is to introduce load where one should strengthen, or to strengthen endlessly where dosed novelty is already possible.

The difference is in what the mode does with novelty. The defensively closed rejects the new. The stabilizing does not yet let it through, but does not reject it. These are not the same. In the closed mode coherence holds precisely through non-admission — the system protects the old reality by letting in nothing that could shake it. In the stabilizing mode coherence grows through accepting conditions — the system says "not now, but I am here," and with each accepted step its capacity increases.

Hence the practical markers that allow them to be told apart in real time. The reaction to support: in the closed mode support is read as misunderstanding ("you don't understand how bad it is"); in the stabilizing mode it is accepted and raises coherence. What happens after a good intervention: in the closed mode — more defense; in the stabilizing — more space. What remains after the session: after a closed one — a repetition of the old position without widening; after a stabilizing one — a little more endurance is added.

A formula worth remembering: defensive closure preserves the old reality; stabilization increases the possibility of future novelty.

This distinction connects directly to the symmetry from Chapter 1. There, perpetual stabilization was named an error — but what was called an error was stabilization that lasts endlessly and leads nowhere. The stabilizing mode in itself is not an error and not a deficiency. It is a full, necessary state of work, in which the system gathers capacity. It becomes an error only when the therapist stays in it forever, having confused the condition of therapy with therapy itself. Stabilization-as-work and stabilization-as-being-stuck can be told apart by one sign only — whether capacity grows over time, or whether it is preserved unchanged.

5.6. Modes shift, and the transitions can be read

Since a mode is a state of the moment, it shifts. And the shifts are not random: transitions have recognizable signs by which the therapist understands that the assembly has moved into another mode, and that something else is now fit.

Coherence is restored, the client is again oriented in body and contact — this is the exit from fragmentation into stabilization. A "maybe" appears, the client for the first time holds an alternative without closing and without collapse — this is the transition from stabilization into exploration. The alternative ceases to be a thought and begins to be experienced, a bodily trace of the new appears — this is the entry into the transitional mode. And in the reverse direction: affect has exceeded coherence, and self, other, or time lose their integrity — this is a breakdown from the transitional mode into fragmentation; an alternative was considered and quickly turned into a threat or was devalued — this is a rollback from exploration into defensive closure; the client stops proving the old reality and says "I can't go there now, but I'm here" — this is a softening from the closed mode into stabilization.

Reading the transitions matters more than naming the modes. The name of a mode is a snapshot. A transition is a movement, and it is the movement that tells the therapist what their last action did to the system. The assembly went into closure after an intervention — this is a strong sign that the intervention was premature or introduced too densely. The assembly moved toward exploration — this is a strong sign that the load fell into the zone of fit. The mode map, in this sense, works together with the formula of Chapter 4: a mode and its shift are the way to see whether an intervention fell into the zone of fit or went beyond it.

5.7. How to determine the mode: by novelty, not by words

The mode map has one practical rule, which is also its main protection against error.

The Cα mode is determined not by what the client says, but by what happens to novelty after its contact with the system.

This matters because words are deceptive. A client may utter "maybe you're right" — and this may be exploration, or it may be defensive closure in which agreement serves as a way to close the topic. A client may be silent — and this may be fragmentation, or it may be a transitional moment in which the new is being experienced for the first time and does not yet have words. Utterances in themselves do not tell the mode. The mode is told by what happened to the new: did it enter, bounce off, scatter the system, or hold for the first time.

Hence a working device. After every significant intervention the therapist can ask themselves: what did my last action do to the client's system? Did more space appear, or more defense? Did coherence rise or fall? Was the new considered, rejected, experienced — or did it destroy the assembly? If the therapist can answer this question, they know the mode. If they cannot, the mode has not yet been read, and the next intervention will rest more on the habit of one's method than on a reading of the moment.

This returns us to where the book began. Premature rightness (Chapter 1) is, in the language of this chapter, an intervention right in content introduced into a mode that cannot take it in: into the defensively closed, where it will strengthen the defense, or into the fragmenting, where it will complete the collapse. Reading the mode is the first and largest filter of fit.

5.8. Where we go next

The Cα mode is the largest distinction of the state of the assembly. It answers the question of what the system is currently doing with novelty: falling apart, closing, assembling, exploring, or letting the new in for the first time. It is the background against which every finer reading of the moment becomes possible.

But the mode does not tell everything. It shows how the system handles the new in general — but does not show how heavily that specific experience we are dealing with weighs. A client may be in the exploratory mode and calmly consider an alternative to one belief — and the same client, in the same mode, will run into another experience that no amount of considering will shift, because for them it is not a thought but reality itself. This weight — the degree to which an experience acts as reality rather than as one of several possible points of view — the mode does not show.

For this a further instrument is needed: the reality weight of experience. On which, Chapter 6. A summary map of the Cα modes, with signs, transitions, and typical errors, is given in the Method Atlas, Appendix B.

Chapter 6. The Reality Weight of Experience

6.1. The person who knows everything and lives the opposite

A client of forty can list every proof that his wife loves him. He does not deny them. Asked directly — "do you know that she loves you?" — he answers "yes, of course I know" and gives examples: how she cares, how she stayed through a hard year, what she says. At the level of knowledge, everything is in place.

And yet every day he experiences himself as unloved. He does not "think" he is unloved — he experiences it. The body is chronically in it: shoulders drawn in, a heaviness in the chest, an apologetic note in the voice. He avoids closeness so as not to confirm a rejection that, as he himself knows, is not there. He tests his wife with questions whose answers he fears in advance. He controls, withdraws, then blames himself for withdrawing. The knowledge that he is loved governs nothing. What governs is the experience that he is unloved.

A therapist who tries to work here with content — to recall the proofs, build the logic, show the distortion — will find that nothing lands. The client will agree with everything and not change one iota. Because the problem is not in what he does not know. The problem is that knowledge and experience have, for him, a different weight as reality. Knowledge weighs little. The experience weighs as if it were the world itself.

This gap — between what the client knows and what is real for them — is recognized by every practitioner. It stands behind the phrases any therapist hears: "I understand I'm not being rejected, but the other's silence is experienced as rejection"; "I know nothing threatens me, but the body lives in threat"; "I understand I have a future, but inside there is no future." In each of these phrases knowledge is not equal to experience. And it is the second that organizes the life.

DDSRF calls what is distinguished here reality weight.

6.2. What reality weight is

Reality weight is the degree to which an experience acts, for the person, as reality. Not how true it is. Not how emotionally strong it is. But how far it organizes the body, attention, expectations, relationships, and the availability of action — even if the person rationally disagrees with it.

This notion resolves the central clinical paradox with which the chapter began.

A client may rationally agree with one thing and experience another as real. Agreement with content changes nothing as long as the reality weight of the old experience remains high.

In the case from 6.1 the knowledge "I am loved" has low reality weight: it is uttered, but organizes neither the body nor action. The experience "I am unloved" has high weight: it holds the body, directs attention, dictates conduct. When we say a client "understands but does not change," we are almost always describing precisely this — the content has shifted, while the reality weight of the old experience has stayed the same.

It is worth connecting this at once to what has already been said. The distinction between "understanding" and "integrating," on which the whole book rests (Chapters 1, 2, 4), gains a scale in the language of this chapter. "To understand" means the content is present with low reality weight. "To integrate" means the new experience's reality weight has grown enough that it has begun to organize experience. Agreement may be an important beginning — but if it stays only content, it does not change reality. Therapy that stops at agreement often stays at the level of RW0–RW1. Therapy that changes a life works with weight: it helps the old reality lose part of its compulsion, and the new experience gather enough weight to become an available alternative. These are different kinds of work, and they are easy to confuse.

6.3. What reality weight is not

Two conflations occur so often that they must be set aside at once — otherwise the notion blurs.

Reality weight is not the same as predictive precision. Predictive activity Pσ — the firmness with which the system holds an expectation, for instance that the other will reject — is one of the layers of the assembly; in Chapter 7 we will see how it can hold a veto. High predictive precision often raises reality weight, and the two are easy to merge. But they are not one. Prediction is only one of the sources of weight. An experience can act as reality even without a strong prediction — through bodily threat, the absence of the other, an old narrative, developmental calibration, life context. Reality weight is an assembly construct: several layers hold it at once. This difference is practical. With a prediction one can sometimes work through an experience that contradicts the expectation. With high reality weight one such experience is usually not enough: the weight is held by several supports, and the work must touch not only the expectation but also the body, the field, the narrative, the calibration, and the context.

Reality weight is not the same as the intensity of affect. This is the same distinction we drew in Chapter 4 between load and intensity, only from the other side. An outwardly weak affect can carry very high reality weight: a quiet, level, almost colorless hopelessness — "I have no future" — can organize a person's entire life without raising its voice. And conversely: a strong emotional storm can have low weight — a flare that thundered and left no trace in how the person experiences themselves afterward. A therapist who orients to the force of affect systematically confuses the loud with the weighty. Weight is read not by loudness but by how far the experience holds the body, directs action, and lets no refutation into itself.

6.4. The five levels of reality weight

Before listing the levels, the main thing about their use must be said. Reality weight always belongs to a specific experience, not to the person as a whole. One cannot say "the client is RW3." One can say only "the experience 'I am unloved' currently has high weight" or "the experience 'if I ask, I'll be humiliated' holds RW3." In one and the same client at one and the same moment, "I am loved" may weigh little, "I am unloved" much, "I can ask" almost nothing, and "if I ask, I'll be humiliated" almost as much as reality itself. So the therapist always specifies: which experience exactly has weight? Without this specification the scale immediately turns into a covert typology — "he's RW4," "she's self-enclosed" — and that is exactly what DDSRF avoids: weight describes the state of an experience in the moment, not a property of the person.

Reality weight is conveniently distinguished at five levels — from an experience that barely organizes experience, to one into which no refutation any longer enters. This is not a ruler with graduations and not a point score; it is five recognizable degrees of how far an experience acts as reality. The level is read, not computed.

RW0 — semantic content. The client can utter a sentence, describe the content, agree with an idea — but it stays words. No bodily trace, no change in action, no presence beyond the conversation. The client speaks of the theme almost as of someone else's; the content changes easily to its opposite without resistance and is quickly forgotten. Example: "Yes, I suppose I deserve love, like everyone" — level, without a pause, without resonance, without a trace in the following minutes. At this level what is usually available is discussion, informing, psychoeducation, clear definitions — what deals with content.

RW1 — a possible perspective. The client admits the idea as one of the possible ones: considers, compares, ponders. There is intellectual interest, but no stable bodily trace yet; the idea is held in conversation but does not govern, and between sessions does not return without a reminder. "I thought about what you said. Maybe I really am too hard on myself. I'm not sure, but I allow it" — the tone level, without a shift. At this level what is usually available is cognitive work, reframing, discussion in the exploratory Cα mode, small behavioral trials.

RW2 — situational reality. The experience becomes real in specific contexts: in some situations it governs, in others not. It is trigger-dependent. Outside the trigger the client speaks of it at a distance, the bodily trace does not appear constantly, and the client can often predict where it will "hit" them. Example: in the office the client speaks calmly about a criticizing boss — but in a meeting in his presence experiences himself as worthless, cannot speak, the body contracts. At this level what is most often fit is work with specific triggers, bodily work at the moment of onset, relational work in the office as a re-enactment, micro-trials in safe contexts.

RW3 — dominant reality. The experience governs the body, attention, and action despite rational disagreement. The client themselves notes the gap — "I understand, but I experience it differently"; the bodily trace is stable or frequently returning; the experience is present in most contexts, not only triggered ones, and directs the choice of relationships, work, behavior. Rational refutation does not enter. This is the level of the client from 6.1. Here arguing with content does not work at all. Here the main question usually becomes the dominant constraint (Chapter 7), and the work goes through a consecutive handling of the layers and through a minimal counter-experience (Chapter 9) whose load carefully matches capacity. What does not work — rational persuasion, presenting contradictory facts, "you know it isn't so," cognitive restructuring without work on the layers.

RW4 — self-enclosed reality. The experience becomes almost impervious to refutation. All incoming data are interpreted in its favor, alternatives do not enter, the system confirms itself. Contradictory facts are reinterpreted to fit the old reality; doubt about the experience does not arise or quickly fades; confirmations are found even where there are none; rational criticism is perceived as a threat. Such a reality has a quality of compulsion. Example: a client is certain his colleagues despise him — and any neutral remark becomes hidden contempt, any support is read as pity ("which is worse"), any absence of reaction as confirmation that he does not deserve attention. At this level direct work with content is not merely useless — it is perceived as an attack. At this level what is usually needed first is stabilization, safety, risk assessment, work with the body and the basic conditions, and where necessary a psychiatric referral. What does not work — argument, proof, insight-work, and in general any intervention that requires the system to be open.

6.5. RW4 and the boundary of safety

RW4 must be addressed separately, because here runs a boundary easy to miss.

High reality weight in itself is not psychosis. RW4 can be a neurotic self-enclosure: a severe shame or paranoid organization in which reality testing is on the whole intact, but one experience has become impervious. Such self-enclosure is worked with cautiously, but it remains psychotherapeutic work.

But if the self-enclosure affects reality testing itself — if it is no longer a matter of an experience weighing heavily, but of the person losing the ability to distinguish it from fact — this is a different zone. On the organization axis discussed later in the book, this is already the area of O4–O5 — a dissociative-fragmented or psychotically disorganizing organization — and here psychiatric and/or specialized clinical assessment is needed. This is the same boundary as in Chapter 7: questions of safety — suicidal risk, psychotic disorganization, severe decompensation — stand above any logic of reading the moment and set the boundary of the work. Reality weight helps see that an experience has become impervious. It does not replace a clinical assessment of whether reality testing is intact.

6.6. How reality weight is read

Reality weight is not computed and not scored in points. It is read — by three markers, each available right in the session.

The first is the bodily trace. Does the experience have a body? Does it change breathing, posture, tone, expression? The more distinctly the experience is present in the body, the higher its reality weight. The knowledge that "everything is fine" often has almost no bodily trace. The experience of threat usually does — sometimes as tension, sometimes as freezing, sometimes as emptiness or loss of access to the body. So the bodily trace is not a standalone criterion: it is read together with action and resistance to refutation, not instead of them.

The second is the effect on action. Does the experience change what the client does or can do? Does it determine choices — whom to avoid, what not to approach, what not to allow oneself? The more the experience governs action, the higher its weight. What weighs little stays words; what weighs much is visible in conduct.

The third is resistance to refutation. What happens when contradictory facts appear? An experience of low weight yields easily to new information. One of high weight does not shift, and sometimes even strengthens, having processed the refutation into its own confirmation. The less effect contradictory data have, the higher the weight.

None of the three markers alone determines the level of weight. A vivid bodily trace without a stable effect on action does not yet mean high weight;

stable avoidance without obvious affect may well mean high weight; and the fact that refutation does not enter is sometimes explained not by weight but by the Cα mode or the layer holding the veto. So weight is read from the whole. An experience that has a stable bodily trace, that governs action, and that lets no refutation into itself is an experience of high reality weight, however calmly the client may speak of it.

6.7. The main rule: weight changes what is possible

From all this follows a rule that connects reality weight to the central formula of the book.

The higher the reality weight of the old configuration, the higher the integration load of any counter-experience — and the more careful the sequence must be.

This is a direct continuation of Chapter 4. The reality weight of the old experience is one of the main factors that raise or lower the load: an intervention harmless at low weight carries, at RW3, an enormous load, because it assaults what for the client is reality itself. Hence the practical consequence behind all the typical errors with this instrument: to treat high weight as low — to argue, persuade, present facts where the experience weighs as world — sharply raises the risk of closing-down or pseudo-agreement. And the reverse is also an error: to conduct deep, multilayered work where simple reframing would suffice, because the weight is in fact not high, is to deepen artificially and lose time.

Reading weight, then, answers not the question "is the client right" but the question "what is at all possible to do with this experience right now." At RW0–RW1, conversation is possible. At RW2, work with triggers and the body in the moment. At RW3, consecutive work on the layers and a minimal counter-experience are needed. At RW4, stabilization and safety come first. A table matching levels to available work is gathered in the Method Atlas (Appendix D); in the main text what matters is the logic, not the grid: the weight of the old sets the requirements for the sequence of steps.

6.8. A practical rule

The whole chapter has one short form worth keeping in mind.

"I understand" is not equal to "this has become reality."

When a client agrees, nods, voices the right thought — this does not mean the experience has changed. It means the content has shifted to RW0–RW1. The old reality with high weight may meanwhile remain untouched, and a week later the client will return exactly where they were — because what changed was words, not weight.

So the therapeutic task is not to obtain agreement with the right content. Agreement may be an important beginning, but in itself it is not equal to a change of weight. The task is to help the new experience gather enough reality weight to become an available alternative to the old reality, and at the same time to let the old reality lose part of its compulsion. This is the real work of change: it does not reduce to content, because the new experience must gather weight through the body, relationships, narrative, and action. How exactly this happens we will come to in Chapter 9.

6.9. Where we go next

We now have two of the three instruments for reading the moment. The Cα mode (Chapter 5) shows what the system does with novelty in general. Reality weight shows how heavily the specific experience we are dealing with weighs — and thereby what is currently possible with it.

But both these instruments describe a state. They tell in which mode the assembly is working and what weight an experience carries — but do not yet tell which layer of the system currently holds the veto on the next step. The client may be in the exploratory mode, the experience may have moderate weight — and still the next step does not land, because it is blocked by the body, or the field, or the life context.

Which layer blocks it and how to determine this is the last of the three instruments for reading the moment. It is the dominant constraint, and it is the subject of the next chapter.

Chapter 7. The Dominant Constraint

7.1. The client who seems "perfectly clear"

A client of thirty comes in with a theme she formulates herself, clearly and at once: "I live in shame. I'm ashamed almost all the time — of what I say, of how I look, of taking up space at all." The request is direct. The shame is visible in every session: in how she apologizes for her tears, how she checks the therapist's face after every sentence, how she breaks off the story about herself mid-word.

The therapist works with the shame. Competently, carefully, within their approach. Names the shame, explores its history, shows its protective function, looks for the early scenes where it formed. The client agrees, weeps, thanks them. And — does not change. Worse: after sessions in which the shame is named directly, she comes in more closed. One day she says: "I understand you want to help. But when you say it, I feel even more ashamed. As if you can see what I'm like."

Here is the key. The shame is active, it is visible, it is stated as the request. But the work with it breaks down not on the shame itself. It breaks down on the fact that in the therapist's presence the shame intensifies — because the therapist is experienced as evaluating, as one more gaze under which the client folds up. Shame is what is visible. But what blocks the work with shame is the field between her and the therapist. As long as the field is experienced as an evaluating gaze, any naming of the shame is the addition of one more gaze. The work must start not with the shame but with how the field is built.

In such work the first step will be not a more accurate naming of the shame but the creation of an experience of small visibility without additional shame. The client must first experience that the therapist can see her and not turn that seeing into evaluation. Only after this will work with the shame become fit. This is what this book calls the question of sequence:

what must become possible earlier so that the next step ceases to be premature.

This difference — between what is visible and what blocks — is the subject of the chapter. Chapter 4 gave the question: when is an intervention fit. This chapter gives an instrument for the reverse side of the same question: what exactly, right now, makes the next step unfit.

7.2. The main question

DDSRF calls what blocks the next step the dominant constraint. It is the layer of the assembly that, at a given moment, holds veto power over change — even if the other layers look ready.

The main question that the dominant constraint seeks runs:

What, right now, has the right to stop change, even if everything else looks ready?

It is worth hearing how this question differs from the usual ones. It is not the question "what is the root of the problem." Not the question "what is the main thing here." Not the question "what does one usually work with in such clients." All three usual questions lead astray — to etiology, to severity, to protocol. The question of the dominant constraint is narrow and practical: what blocks the next concrete step.

In most working moments it is useful to look for one layer through which to begin. Sometimes the veto is held by a pair of layers bound together — for example, body and thresholds, field and old calibration, life-world and bodily exhaustion. But even then the task is not to declare "everything affects everything," but to find the nearest node, work with which will open the next step. And this is good news for practice: at any moment, however complex the client, there is usually one place, work with which opens movement, and bypassing which makes precisely this next step premature.

To find this layer is the central methodological task of reading the moment. A therapist who can find the veto gains one of the main orienting points for reading the moment. A therapist who does not look for it risks working with the right content in the wrong place — even when their interventions are right in content. This is a direct continuation of Chapter 1: premature rightness is most often work with the right content while bypassing the layer that holds the veto.

7.3. Three statuses of a layer

Before looking for the veto, one must distinguish three different statuses any layer of the assembly can be in. They are confused constantly, and from that confusion comes much of the work that stalls.

The **active layer** is the layer that participates in the current assembly and is visible in the session. The shame of the client from 7.1 is an active layer. It is on the surface, it is stated, it colors every remark. The typical error with the active layer is to follow the most vivid material simply because it is most vivid.

The **load-bearing layer** is the layer that substantially supports the current configuration. Without it the configuration does not hold. The load-bearing layer is not always visible; sometimes it works quietly, and that is exactly why it is missed. The typical error with the load-bearing layer is to assume that since a layer supports the configuration, it is the one to start with; supporting the configuration and being the point of entry into the work are not the same thing.

The **layer with veto power** is the layer that blocks the next step of change. Until work with it has begun, other steps do not land. In the case of the client from 7.1 the veto is held by the field — the layer of the other — and not at all by the shame, which is active and visible. The typical error with the veto layer is to bypass it: to work to one side of the very thing that makes the next step premature.

These are three different questions, and they cannot be reduced to one another. The active layer answers "what is visible." The load-bearing — "what holds." The veto — "what blocks." One and the same layer may simultaneously be active, load-bearing, and hold the veto — but this cannot be assumed in advance, it must be read. A therapist who automatically works with what is most visibly active very often misses: the most noticeable thing in a client's material rarely coincides with what blocks movement. Distinguishing these three statuses is the first skill of reading the dominant constraint. In the Method Atlas it is gathered into the working table of the dominant constraint protocol (Appendix C).

7.4. The seven layers where a veto can live

A veto can be held by any of the seven layers of the assembly. Below — each layer and how the veto is recognized on it specifically. These are not diagnostic categories and not client types. They are places where a block may, at a given moment, be located. In the same client at different moments the veto may shift from one layer to another.

Body, B(t). The veto is here when the client "understands everything," but the body does not follow the understanding. Signs: disturbed sleep, exhaustion, chronic pain, autonomic dysregulation. One of the strongest markers of a body veto: after bodily regulation — sleep, rest, breathing, sometimes medical correction — availability for all the rest of the work rises sharply. While the veto is with the body, interpretation, exposure, work with meaning, and the demand for action are premature. Sleep, regulation, bodily stability, and where necessary medical assessment must come first.

The other and the field, S(t). The veto is here when the intervention breaks down not on content but on relationship. A neutral question is experienced as evaluation, a pause as rejection, involvement as intrusion. This is the veto of the client from 7.1. While the veto is with the field, the disclosure of shame, deep interpretation, and attachment work are premature. The attunement of the field must come first: safety of visibility, repair of contact, restoration of the experience that one is not being evaluated here.

Narrative, N(t). The veto is here when any new experience is absorbed by the old story. Whatever happens, it is built into the former plot: "it's always like this with me," "this changes nothing," "this is a fluke." The old story works as a funnel in which the new loses the status of new. While the veto is with the narrative, behavioral experiments without symbolic processing are premature — the client will run the experiment and write its result into the same story. A weakening of the old narrative must come first: a new language, a new frame in which the new experience can hold as new.

Predictive precision, Pσ. The veto is here when contradictory facts do not update experience. Ambiguous signals are read steadily in one direction — as threat, as shame, as rejection — and refuting data do not change this reading. This is the layer on which rational dissuasion breaks down: arguing with the belief is useless, because the problem is not in the content of the belief but in the fact that the system predicts with such certainty that the data do not get through. A lowering of the precision of the old prediction must come first — but not through argument, through the body, the field, and repeated experience that accumulates below the threshold of the argument.

Thresholds of coherence, Θ. The veto is here when, on approaching the material, coherence falls. On approaching the theme the client loses the thread, drops into emptiness, into derealization, into panic; speech breaks off or drifts into abstraction. This is not resistance and not unwillingness — it is the system's defense against collapse. While the veto is with the thresholds, transformational work, traumatic material, and strong confrontation are premature. A restoration of coherence must come first: small doses of material, titration, work at the edge and not beyond it.

Developmental calibration, D_cal. The veto is here when the present is experienced as an old situation. The reaction is clearly larger than the event; "then" automatically organizes "now." The client reacts to today's person or today's situation by the measure of a long-ago scene, and this calibration works independently of their understanding. While the veto is with the calibration, work only with the current event is premature — it does not reach what organizes the reaction. A recognition of the old calibration and a distinction between "then" and "now" must come first.

The life-world, Λ. The veto is here when the real environment keeps producing threat. Violence at home, exhausting work, poverty, humiliation, legal uncertainty — external conditions that nullify any inner work. This is the layer that internally-oriented therapists miss most often. While the veto is with the life-world, inner work without a change of conditions is premature — and worse, can intensify the sense of personal inadequacy, because the client "works on themselves" while the conditions keep destroying. A change of conditions must come first: protection, resources, legal or social help.

The seven layers are not a sequence and not a hierarchy. They are a map of places. At each moment the veto may be held by one layer or a pair of layers bound together. The task is to determine where exactly the veto runs right now, and not by eye.

7.5. Frequent confusions of the veto

The seven layers are described separately, but in living work neighboring layers are easily confused. Four pairs are confused most often, and it is worth knowing how they differ.

Field and calibration — S(t) or D_cal. In both cases the other is experienced through an old threat, and the two pictures look alike: the client is on guard, expects evaluation, defends. The difference is in where the next step is currently blocked. If it is precisely the current encounter with this therapist that makes the material non-integrable — the field, S(t), is more likely. If the reaction is steadily carried across different relationships and situations, while the current contact is in itself stable enough — the old calibration, D_cal, is more likely.

Body and thresholds — B(t) or Θ. Both pictures look like a drop in the capacity to work. What helps tell them apart is what restores availability. With a body veto, work becomes more available after bodily stabilization: sleep, rest, regulation, medical correction. With a threshold veto the main sign is different — coherence falls precisely on approaching the material, even when the basic body is relatively stable.

Narrative and predictive precision — N(t) or Pσ. In both cases the new experience does not enter. But it fails to enter in different ways. The narrative absorbs the new experience into the old story: the event happens, but its meaning is rewritten to fit the former plot. Predictive precision does not let the data update the expectation: the event does not even reach meaning, because it is read in advance. In the first case a new language and a new frame must come first. In the second — repeated experience that gradually lowers the precision of the old expectation.

The life-world and inner organization — Λ or the inner layers. When work stalls, it is easy to attribute this to the client's inner assembly — to "resistance," to defense, to immaturity. The life-world veto is recognized where the office creates clarity and the life environment systematically nullifies it: the client composes themselves in the session and returns to conditions that destroy them again. Here the matter is not the inner assembly but the fact that the external world really keeps producing threat.

In Appendix C these distinctions are gathered into a working table for supervision and case formulation.

7.6. Three tests: how to determine the veto, not by eye

A single indicator is a hypothesis, not a conclusion. The client sleeps badly — a hypothesis about the body. The client withdraws in contact — a hypothesis about the field. A hypothesis becomes a working one only through triangulation: when at least two independent sources point to the same layer. For this there are three tests, and they have different strengths.

Test 1. The failure test. The question: which correct interventions are already failing to land or are strengthening the defense? This is the strongest test, because it rests on what has already been observed, not on the imagined. If the client understands, agrees, but nothing changes — the veto is probably with the body, predictive precision, or calibration. If they withdraw specifically in contact — probably with the field. If any new thought becomes part of the old story — with the narrative. If coherence falls on approaching the theme — with the thresholds. If therapy works in the session but life outside the door nullifies it all — with the life-world. The failure test is read directly from what has already happened in the work.

Test 2. The small-support test. The question: which small shift immediately raises coherence or opens access to the work? Almost as strong as the first, because it too rests on an observed effect. If sleep, grounding, breathing, or rest sharply raise the capacity to work — the veto is with the body. If the sentence "we can go more slowly" returns the client to contact — with the field or the thresholds. If a new formulation of the story gives space — with the narrative. If a change of real conditions gives more than any interpretation — with the life-world.

Test 3. The counterfactual test. The question: if this layer were temporarily stabilized, would the next step become possible? If yes — it is a candidate for the dominant constraint. If no — the layer is important but does not hold the veto. Example: a client in shame, and it seems one should work with the shame. But if one imagines the shame slightly lowered — the work is still impossible, because the client has not slept for three months and the body is wrecked. So right now the veto is with the body, not the shame.

The third test has an important weakness, and it must be known. The counterfactual test is easily infected by the therapist's preferences. A body-oriented therapist will imagine that what should be stabilized is the body; a psychoanalyst — the transference; a cognitive therapist — the belief. The imagined experiment is too pliable to what the therapist knows how to work with. So the third test is applied last — after the two tests that rest on the observed, and as a check, not in their place.

7.7. The rule of triangulation

Hence a rule that separates a working hypothesis from a guess.

A veto hypothesis counts as strong only if at least two independent tests point to one layer.

If only the counterfactual test pointed to the layer — the hypothesis is weak. If the counterfactual plus one clinical indicator — medium. If at least two of the three tests converge — strong. It is worth working on a strong hypothesis. A weak one — do not discard, but do not turn into a plan of work either: add information, observe, check again.

This is not bureaucracy and not pseudo-science. It is protection against the most frequent error in reading the moment — seeing the veto where one knows how to work. Triangulation forces the hypothesis through two independent observations, and thereby tears it away from the therapist's preferences.

There is also an additional check, especially useful in supervision: the advocate of another school. The question: which layer would a specialist of a different orientation call dominant? Each school has its habitual entry — the layer it notices first, because it knows how to work with it. One approach sees the body first, another the transference, a third the schema, a fourth the thresholds, a fifth the environment. This is not a defect of the schools; it is their specialization. But precisely for this reason the question "what would a colleague of a different orientation see?" lowers the blindness of one's own school. If all the alternative views converge on one layer — the triangulation is strong. If they diverge — a more careful reading is needed, and the habitual layer of one's own school becomes the first candidate for reconsideration, not for confirmation.

7.8. Three distinctions that decide everything

Three reading errors occur so often and cost so much that they are worth naming separately.

The deep source is not the same as the veto now. The dominant constraint is not the root of the problem. It is what blocks the next step. They may coincide, but often they do not. A client may have a deep developmental trauma — that is the root. But right now he is not sleeping, is overloaded, is in autonomic dysregulation. Work with the trauma will be premature not because the trauma is unimportant, but because the veto is currently held by the body. After the body is stabilized the veto will shift, and then the calibration will become the next dominant constraint. But not before. To treat the "root" while bypassing the current veto is a direct path to fragmentation or closing-down.

What is most visible is not the same as the veto now. The most vivid thing in a client's material is often not what blocks movement. The shame of the client from 7.1 was the most vivid — and was an active layer, not a veto layer. The veto was held by the field. A therapist who follows the vividness of the material systematically works with the wrong layer. Vividness is a property of the active layer. Blocking is a property of the veto layer. These are different things, and a session that stalls under correct interventions is almost always a sign that they have been confused.

Clinical importance is not the same as the dominant constraint. Material may be very important and still not block the next step. And conversely: a layer may seem secondary, yet it is the one that makes the next step impossible. Importance and veto are different axes, and they cannot be identified with each other. This distinction has a boundary that must be named plainly. Questions of safety stand above the logic of the veto altogether. Suicidal risk, violence, psychotic disorganization, medical danger, severe dissociation — these are not candidates for "the dominant constraint" that other layers compete with. They are a clinical priority that sets the boundary of the work and temporarily suspends the usual method of reading the moment. The dominant constraint is an instrument for the space between the extremes spoken of in Chapter 2. Where safety is at stake, what operates is not the logic of the veto but responsibility for life and the corresponding help.

7.9. The veto shifts: it is a hypothesis about a step, not a diagnosis

The dominant constraint is not static. It shifts as the work proceeds, and this is its nature, not a flaw.

The rhythm of the work is this. Determine the current veto through triangulation. Work with it — not ignoring the other layers, but giving priority to what blocks. When the veto lowers, check anew: which layer now blocks the next step? The new dominant constraint may turn out to be a quite different layer than the previous one.

There is a second reason the veto is not static: it depends not only on the client but on which step exactly we are about to take. The dominant constraint is always determined relative to the next step. One cannot say "the client has a veto in the body" in general. More precisely: "for work with traumatic material the veto is currently in the body." For another step — say, a simple reflection of the state — that same body may hold no veto at all. So the formulation of the veto must always include not only the layer but the step that this layer makes premature. The same moment has different dominant constraints for different interventions.

This does not mean "go through all the layers in turn" — there is no such plan, because it is not known in advance where the veto will shift. It means something else: the dominant constraint is a working hypothesis about the next step, not a diagnosis of a layer. A therapist who found the veto once and works with it for months, without checking whether it has shifted, makes the same error as one who never looked for it. The veto is something to re-read, not something determined once.

And one more consequence, important for case formulation. The dominant constraint is formulated concretely, not in a single word. "Trauma," "shame," "attachment" — these are not formulations of the veto, they are names of layers or themes. A strong formulation names the layer, its current state, and what is premature because of it: for example, "the veto is in the body — autonomic hypoactivation against a background of several months without proper sleep; until basic regulation is restored, work with traumatic material will be premature." Such a formulation contains at once both the hypothesis and its clinical consequence. How this enters the one-page case formulation we return to in the Method Atlas (Appendices A and C).

7.10. A practical check

The dominant constraint has a simple check of working accuracy that requires neither theory nor agreement with DDSRF.

The dominant constraint has been found when working with it increases the possibility of the next step, and bypassing it makes the next step premature.

This is not a philosophical assumption but a clinical observation available in the session itself. If the veto hypothesis hit the right layer — space appears in the work: the client becomes more available, the next step lands, movement resumes. If the hypothesis missed — no space appears, however right the interventions may be in content. And then what is needed is not a stronger intervention but a different veto hypothesis.

In this sense the dominant constraint is a self-correcting instrument. It does not prove itself once and for all. It makes the therapist watch: did more space for the next step appear after working with this layer. If it did — the hypothesis is probably right. If not — the hypothesis is reconsidered. At the same time the absence of space does not by itself unambiguously refute the hypothesis: work with a correctly found veto may fail for other reasons too — a weak intervention, a thin field, an overloaded therapist, a changed context. So the instrument is not proving but precisely correcting: it keeps the therapist in constant re-reading rather than delivering a final verdict. This returns us to the central formula of Chapter 4: an intervention becomes fit when its load falls into the zone of fit. The dominant constraint is what most often holds the boundary of the zone. To find the veto is to find where the boundary of the currently-fit runs.

7.11. Where we go next

We now have three instruments for reading the moment. The Cα mode shows what the system does with novelty. Reality weight shows how far an experience acts as reality. The dominant constraint shows which layer currently holds veto power over the next step.

Together they make the formula of Chapter 4 practically applicable. We can now ask not only “is the intervention right” but “does it fall into the current zone of fit.” We can see when the system explores and when it defends;

when an experience has too much weight to be contested; and which layer makes the next step premature.

But the main practical question remains. If the next step is premature now — what must become possible earlier?

This is the question of sequence, and it will be the subject of the next chapter. The principle of sequence connects everything already built: integrative capacity, the Cα mode, reality weight, and the dominant constraint. It turns the reading of the moment into a clinical decision. The dominant constraint says where the veto currently runs. The principle of sequence says how to work with that veto so that change becomes possible.

Part III

Change, Application, and Boundaries

Chapter 8. The Principle of Sequence

8.1. The same steps, a different order

Return to the client from Chapter 7 — the one who lives in shame, who declares shame as the request, and with whom work on the shame breaks down because the veto holds the field: the therapist is experienced as one more appraising gaze.

Suppose the therapist has read everything correctly. He knows several things are needed. The client needs to live through an experience of being seen without being judged — that she can be seen and not condemned. The shame needs to be named in a way that does not add yet another gaze. The early scenes where the shame took shape need to be reached. Something, perhaps, needs to change in how she presents herself to the world. All of these are the right steps. Not one of them is wrong in content.

And everything depends on the order. If the therapist begins by naming the shame, he adds a gaze, and the field closes; everything else becomes unavailable. If he begins with the early scenes, he leads the client into high-weight material while the field does not yet hold, and she either closes down or fragments. If he begins with how she presents herself to the world, he demands action from a system that has not yet lived through the safety of being seen even in the consulting room. In this assembly the fitting order begins with one thing: to create an experience of being seen without judgment in the room itself. Until that exists, everything else is premature. When it exists, the next step opens — and only then does it become visible which step it is.

This is the subject of the chapter. The right steps are not enough. Between a set of right steps and change stands the order. The same work, carried out in one sequence, lands and changes; carried out in another, it closes the system down, fragments it, or yields nothing. Order is not an organizational detail. It is a clinical variable in its own right, and this chapter is about how to read it.

8.2. The principle of sequence

Everything built in the previous chapters converges on a single principle.

> A clinically right action becomes fit only in the order in which the client's system, the therapist, and the field can integrate it.

This is not a fourth instrument for reading the moment. It is the grammar that ties the formula of fit and the three reading instruments into a clinical decision. Chapter 4 gave the concept of fit. Chapters 5, 6, and 7 gave three ways to read the state of the assembly. The principle of sequence answers the question that arises the moment all of this has been read: in what order to bring in what must be brought in?

And this principle inverts the usual logic. Clinical thinking usually asks: what is central here, where to begin, what is the root. The principle of sequence asks differently. Not "what is most important," but "what must become possible earlier, so that the important can land at all." The most important thing often stands last in the order, not first — because it carries the highest load and requires that much become possible before it.

Sequence operates at different scales. Within a single utterance: to say it now or to stay silent. Within a session: first to restore coherence or to go straight to the material. Within months of work: first the field, then the shame, then the early scenes, then action in the world. The scales differ, but the question at each is the same: what must become possible earlier?

8.3. The main question: what must become possible earlier

The whole book has one question it has been moving toward since the first chapter. It sounded in advance in the discussion of premature rightness, then in the formula of fit, then in the work with the veto. Now it becomes the central methodological question of practice.

What must become possible earlier?

This question is asked whenever the needed next step turns out to be premature. It does not ask "how to force the step to land," and it does not ask "whether to abandon the step." It asks a third thing: what smaller step must happen first, so that the needed one stops being premature.

For the client in 8.1, the needed step is work on the shame. It is premature. The question "what must become possible earlier" gives the answer: an experience of being seen without judgment. That is the preceding term of the sequence. And if even that is impossible now, the question is asked again, of it: what must become possible earlier, so that even the experience of being seen becomes available? Perhaps a minimal steadiness of the field. Perhaps simply that the client lives through the therapist not flinching from the first thing she said. The question can be asked recursively until a step is found that is available now. That is where the sequence begins.

This inverts the direction of clinical planning. Not "here is the goal, we go to it in a straight line," but "here is the goal, and back from it — what must stand before it, and before what stands before that, until we reach what is possible today." A sequence is built from the end and carried out from the beginning. This does not mean the therapist knows the whole path in advance. He knows only the nearest needed step that is premature now, and looks for the condition without which that step will not land; the rest of the path shows itself as the work moves.

In live work this sounds like a simple chain of questions. What step seems clinically needed? Why is it premature now? What must become possible earlier, so that it stops being premature? What still smaller step is available today? What will change in the system if it happens? This is not a checklist and not an algorithm — it is a grammar of order. It is there so that the therapist does not jump from the goal straight to the intervention, bypassing the conditions without which that intervention will not land.

8.4. How the three instruments converge on one order

The principle of sequence adds no new reading. It uses the three that already exist — the Cα mode, reality weight, the dominant constraint — and brings them together into one answer about order.

They work not in turn but together, and each is responsible for its own part of the question about the next step. The Cα mode says whether the system can take in anything new at all right now, or whether it is closed, fragmenting, only stabilizing. Reality weight says what load this particular experience carries — whether it can be touched with a word or whether it weighs as world. The dominant constraint says which layer holds the veto and must therefore be addressed before the rest.

Bring this together on the client in 8.1. The dominant constraint points to the field: the veto is there. The Cα mode at the moment of naming the shame is defensively closed: the system does not let it through. The reality weight of the experience "if I am seen, I will be destroyed" is high, RW3: for her this is not a thought but reality. The three readings converge on a single conclusion about order: the first term of the sequence can be neither an interpretation of the shame (it will run into the closed mode), nor the early scenes (they will run into the high weight), nor a demand for action (it will run into the veto of the field). The first can only be what works directly on the veto layer at minimal load: a small experience of being seen without judgment that the field is able to let through. The three instruments did not give three different answers. They converged on one, and that convergence is the sequence, read.

This is the sense of what was said at the close of Chapter 7: the dominant constraint says where the veto runs, and the principle of sequence says how to work with that veto so that change becomes possible. The reading gives a point. The sequence gives a direction and the order of steps out from it.

8.5. Sequence is not a plan and not a protocol

Here the same caution is needed as with the dominant constraint: a sequence is not a route drawn up in advance.

One cannot write out "first the field, then the shame, then the early scenes, then action" as a six-month plan. Because every step taken changes the system, and the next term of the sequence becomes visible only after the previous one has happened. When the client's field begins to hold being-seen without judgment, the veto will shift — and only then will it become clear what now blocks the next step. Perhaps it will turn out to be reality weight. Perhaps a bodily dysregulation that was not visible behind the field before. Perhaps something in the life context. This is not known in advance.

So a sequence is not built once. It is re-specified at every step, exactly as the veto is re-read in Chapter 7. The principle of sequence is not an algorithm that issues a route, but a way of asking, each time: what is available now, and what will that make possible next. The therapist holds in mind not a written-out plan but one live question, asked anew after each shift.

From this follows how sequence relates to the phase models familiar from various schools. A phase model usually sets a general macro-logic of order: first stabilization, then processing, then integration. This is a useful clinical discipline, especially in trauma therapy, and within their phases good phase approaches also read the client's state. But a phase model remains a general frame. The principle of sequence works at a different level: it derives the order from a reading of a particular assembly at a particular moment. Sometimes that derivation will coincide with phase logic. Sometimes it will call for a different move. Sequence does not argue with phase models; it explains why they work when they work, and gives a way to read order where no ready phase scheme exists.

8.6. Two errors of order

Sequence has two characteristic errors, and both were already named in Chapter 1. Now it can be seen that both are errors precisely of order.

The first is too early. This is premature rightness: a right step brought in before what should have become possible earlier has become possible. The therapist saw the goal and went to it in a straight line, bypassing the intermediate terms of the sequence. The step was right — but not at this place in the order. The result is closing-down, fragmentation, or pseudo-agreement. In the language of this chapter, premature rightness is a violation of order forward: a step taken before its place.

The second is never. This is perpetual stabilization: the therapist endlessly prepares the ground and never takes the next step, even when the sequence already allows it. Here the violation of order is the reverse — the step is not taken although its place in the sequence has already come. The field already holds, the weight has already dropped, the mode is already exploratory — and the therapist keeps reinforcing and stabilizing, having confused the condition for the work with the work itself. The system freezes in a readiness that leads nowhere.

These two errors are symmetrical, and the principle of sequence is what holds the space between them. It demands two different things at once: the patience not to go forward before the place, and the resolve not to get stuck once the place has come. Neither caution by itself nor courage by itself gives the right sequence. Only a reading of which step is now in its place gives it.

8.7. Sequence is dyadic

Everything said about sequence on the client's side is true for the other two participants as well — the therapist and the field. The order must be one that all three can withstand.

It happens that the sequence is clear on the client's side but does not hold on the therapist's. The next step requires the therapist to stay with the client's rage, or with his devaluation, or with his own helplessness — and the therapist has not yet reached that step in his own sequence. Then a step that is right for the client is premature for the dyad: the field on the therapist's side will not withstand it. This is a direct consequence of the dyadic formula of Chapter 4 — fit requires that the load be held by all three. A sequence, then, has not one thread but three, and one can move only where they coincide.

Sometimes the work consists precisely in advancing the therapist's sequence, or the field's, rather than the client's. The therapist, in supervision, builds capacity for what he cannot yet withstand. The field, over the course of the work, gradually becomes denser, and what was premature in a thin field becomes possible in a dense one. The client's sequence sometimes waits for the other two to catch up. This is not delay and not resistance — it is part of the same reading of order.

And the sequence is not sealed inside the consulting room. Sometimes its first step lies not in the meeting but in a change of life conditions — in protection, in the reduction of external load, in legal or social help. If the life-world keeps destroying the system (a veto on Λ, Chapter 7), dyadic work can be entirely right and still fail to hold, because the environment zeroes it out faster than it gains weight. Then the first term of the sequence is outside the room, and to recognize this is also part of the reading of order.

8.8. Where we go next

The principle of sequence completes the core of clinical reading and order. We have the concept of fit (Chapter 4), three instruments for reading the moment (Chapters 5, 6, 7), and a grammar of order that ties them into a decision (this chapter). Together they answer the question with which the book began: how not to be prematurely right — and how, at the same time, not to get stuck in endless preparation.

But one question remains open. Sequence leads step by step to the moment where change can truly begin — to the moment when the new stops being preparation and is experienced, for the first time, as reality. What exactly happens in that moment? How does it differ from insight, from understanding, from agreement? How does a new experience gain the very reality weight without which change does not hold?

This is the moment of counter-experience. Sequence leads to it; reality weight explains why it is needed; the Cα mode says when it is possible. But the moment itself has not yet been described. Here the book moves from the core of reading and order to the core of change: the next chapter is about the very moment when the new is first experienced as reality, and about what distinguishes a change in the availability of the territory from a mere change of the map. This is Chapter 9 — the minimal counter-experience and ICAE.

Chapter 9. The Minimal Counter-Experience and ICAE

9.1. Two conversations about the same thing

The client we worked with in Chapters 7 and 8 — the one who lives in shame, with whom the veto held the field. Suppose the sequence has done its work: the field has come to hold being-seen, and one day in a session this happens.

First version. The client says: "I've understood. My shame is a defense. As a child I was constantly being judged, and I learned to hide so as not to be condemned. Now I understand where it comes from." She speaks calmly, coherently, precisely. It is a correct formulation — perhaps the very one the therapist has been leading her toward for months. She nods, thanks him, says it has become clearer to her. A week later she comes in exactly as she was.

Second version. The client tells something about herself — small, but something she used to be ashamed of. She says it and catches herself, waiting for the therapist's reaction. The therapist does not flinch, does not judge, simply stays beside her. And the client suddenly falls silent, breathes a little differently, and says: "Strange. I just said something, and… nothing happened. You didn't turn away." Her voice trembles. This is not a formulation and not an understanding. It is something that happened — for the first time. A week later she recalls this moment on her own and says that at work, once, she was able not to hide.

In the first version the client received an insight. In the second she lived through a counter-experience. And these are not two degrees of the same thing. They are two different things, and the difference between them is the center of the whole theory of change in this book.

9.2. Insight changes the map, counter-experience changes the availability of the territory

Insight is a shift in understanding. The client sees, recognizes, formulates, connects. He gains a more accurate map of his reality: where the shame came from, how the defense is built, what the symptom means. Insight works with the map.

Counter-experience is a shift in lived possibility. The client does not understand differently — he experiences differently. He does, or finds himself in, what the old configuration counted as impossible or dangerous — and lives through the fact that it happened and he was not destroyed. Counter-experience works not with the map but with the availability of the territory.

Insight changes the map. Counter-experience changes the availability of the territory.

This distinction explains one of the most frequent disappointments in practice: the client has understood everything, formulates more precisely than the therapist, agrees with every interpretation — and does not change. Because understanding the right idea is not the same as integrating it. A map of any precision does not make available a territory that is experienced as closed. A therapist who works only at the level of insight can spend months gaining ever clearer "agreement" without a single real shift. And a therapist who has noticed and held one small counter-experience can lay the beginning of structural change — because for the first time it was not the map that changed but what had become livably possible for the client.

This is the culmination of a distinction that has run through the whole book. "To understand" and "to integrate" (Chapters 1, 2, 4), knowledge and lived reality, low and high reality weight (Chapter 6) — all of it is about one thing. Insight changes the content. Counter-experience gives the new content a chance to gain reality weight. It is precisely through repeated counter-experiences that a new experience gradually acquires the weight without which, as we saw in Chapter 6, change does not hold.

Here two notions that are easily merged must be separated at once. Not every counter-experience immediately becomes an ICAE. A counter-experience is a moment of other lived possibility. ICAE is the case in which the possibility did not merely flicker but was held long enough and began to enter the body, the relationship, the narrative, and action. So in this chapter we first distinguish insight from counter-experience, and then a plain counter-experience from an integrated one — that is, ICAE. We will return to the term itself and its expansion below, when we come to the two axes.

9.3. What a minimal counter-experience is

A counter-experience that actually integrates is almost always minimal. It is the smallest experience of a different organization of reality that already differs from the old configuration enough to begin weakening it, but does not yet exceed the current integrative capacity enough to provoke defensive closure, fragmentation, or devaluation.

The key word is minimal, and it is easily misread. Minimality is not absolute. It is always relative to a particular client, a particular moment, the current Cα mode, and the coherence threshold. For one client a minimal counter-experience is to raise their eyes to the therapist for two seconds. For another, to speak before a group. For a third, to say aloud "I am in pain." What is a momentous step for one is routine for another. Minimality is read not by the size of the action but by its relation to the system's current capacity.

This continues directly from the formula of fit in Chapter 4. A minimal counter-experience is a counter-experience whose load falls into the zone of fit: enough for the new to begin, not so much that the system closes down. Too small a step shifts nothing. Too large a one does not land. The minimal counter-experience is the zone found between them, translated from reading into action.

9.4. How to recognize a counter-experience

A counter-experience is easily confused with things that resemble it — with a strong emotion, with an insight, with a good session. So it is worth knowing its signs. The full list of eight criteria is gathered in the Method Atlas (Appendix F); here I will name the six main ones. The other two — relative minimality and correspondence to the current Cα mode — were already introduced in the previous section and in Chapter 5.

The first and decisive one: a counter-experience is lived, not explained. It has a "happened," not only a "saw." Not "I understood that I am not rejected," but "I said something vulnerable and was not rejected." If the client's report contains only a new understanding and no event that occurred, it is an insight, not a counter-experience.

The second: a counter-experience has a bodily trace. Even a small one — the breathing changed, the shoulders let go, contact was held longer, a micro-pause appeared, a tightening went. The bodily trace need not be only breath or relaxation: sometimes it is a pause, a slowing, less tightening, the appearance of support, silence instead of the former mobilization, or a first access to the body after its absence. If the new experience left no bodily or regulatory trace at all — not even the smallest — it is, most likely, an insight. The body is the first sign by which a counter-experience differs from a thought about it.

The third: a counter-experience does not attack the old reality head-on. If the old configuration says "being seen is dangerous," the counter-experience is not the refutation "being seen is safe, trust me." It is a small fact of something lived: "I was a little bit visible and did not fall apart." Not a conviction and not a proof, but an event the old configuration cannot wholly absorb. A direct refutation the old reality often reprocesses into its own confirmation; a small lived fact is harder for it to absorb at once.

The fourth, closely linked: a counter-experience does not raise the reality weight of the old configuration. This is a subtle and important point. It happens that a technically positive intervention strengthens precisely the old. Praise to a shame-bound client not infrequently raises the weight of "I am being judged," because it is experienced as one more act of appraisal. On the surface — support. In essence — reinforcement of the old reality. A counter-experience is checked not by whether it was pleasant but by whether the old configuration weakened or strengthened after it. And here it is important not to confuse a short-term activation of the old configuration with a strengthening of its weight. After a real counter-experience the old reality may rise for a time: the client takes fright at the new, rolls back, feels shame again. This does not yet mean the counter-experience was false. The dangerous sign is different — when after the intervention the old configuration becomes more convincing, more sealed, gains new confirmation. Then it was not a counter-experience but a reinforcement of the old.

The fifth: a counter-experience is potentially repeatable. If the experience is possible only in a unique dramatic moment and has no path to repetition, it may be a strong session but not the beginning of structural change. Without the possibility of repetition there is no accumulation, and change, as we will see, holds precisely on accumulation.

There is also a sixth sign, which stands apart: a counter-experience can usually be named by the client in their own words — not at once and not precisely, but somehow. “Strange, but I didn’t fall through”; “I managed a little”; “there’s a bit more room.” If the experience left no trace in speech at all, it risks not integrating. The words need not be accurate — but a counter-experience usually finds them.

9.5. Two axes: what happened and how far it took hold

Here a distinction must be introduced that saves one from the most frequent error in working with change. There are two different questions about any counter-experience, and they are constantly confused.

The first question: what happened in the moment? This is the micro-dynamics. The client may simply receive an explanation (not yet change). He may live through a shift of state — it became easier, warmer, clearer (real, but it may vanish by evening). He may live through a first small counter-experience — a patch of different reality. He may hold it at once through several channels — body, relationship, narrative, action. This is ICAE — the Integrated Counter-Attractor Experience: the moment when a new possibility did not merely flicker but was lived and held. It is one of the most significant kinds of shift that can occur in a single session.

The second question is entirely different: how far did it take hold over time? This is durability. It is one thing to experience differently once in a session. Another, to be able to summon that experience deliberately. A third, when the old configuration has weakened and the new has become comparably available. A fourth, when the new organization of experience has become part of ordinary life, not an event in the consulting room.

These are two different axes, and they cannot be collapsed. A strong session answers the first question. Structural change answers the second. Between “an ICAE happened in the room today” and “the client’s life has changed” lie weeks or months of work. A therapist who confuses these axes takes a vivid session for recovery — and is then puzzled why a week later the client is "as he was." He is not as he was: one counter-experience took place. But one counter-experience is an event on the first axis, not an achievement on the second. Both scales — the micro-dynamics of integration and the durability of change — are set out in the Method Atlas (Appendix G); for practice what matters most is to hold the fact itself, that these are two different questions.

9.6. Change goes through oscillations

From here comes the most important thing to know about how change proceeds. It does not go in a straight line. It goes through oscillations between the old configuration and the new counter-experience.

The typical picture looks like this. In a session the client lives through safe visibility — a real ICAE, held through the body and contact. Between sessions the old reality takes over again: she remembers the relief but lives again in shame. In the next session she lives through a small counter-experience again. After several such cycles there appears an ability to summon the new experience beyond the room as well. The old does not leave at once — it has years and decades of history, and one episode of the new cannot instantly displace it.

This must be said plainly, because on it depends whether the therapist destroys his own work. A rollback after a counter-experience is not a failure and not proof that the counter-experience was false. It is the normal form of the movement of integration. A therapist who, at the first rollback, decides it "didn't work" and changes tactics cuts off the very oscillation that is the mechanism of consolidation. A rollback by itself is not a signal to change course; often it is part of the course. But its character must be read: if rollbacks become deeper, more dangerous, or last longer, this is no longer normal oscillation but a reason to reconsider the load, the field, or the sequence.

What, then, tells us that change is really consolidating? Not the presence of rollbacks — they are usually to be expected — but a change in their character. Three things. First: the speed of return — if before, after a rollback, the client returned to the new experience over weeks, now it is days, then hours. Second: the breadth of transfer — the new experience appears no longer only in the room but first with intimates, then with strangers, then on its own. Third: the waning power of the old — the old reality still rises but no longer seizes the whole; the client notices the old experience without getting lost in it. By these three signs consolidation can be seen that is invisible if one looks only at the presence or absence of breakdowns.

9.7. The real counter-experience and its look-alikes

Counter-experience has several convincing look-alikes. If they are not distinguished, therapy can move in the wrong direction for months.

Catharsis. A strong affective discharge — tears, rage, a breakthrough — that feels like a huge event and leaves no trace in how the client experiences himself afterward. A week later, all as it was. The force of affect does not equal a counter-experience: a storm may rage through without shifting anything, while a quiet moment of "I said it and was not rejected" may shift it. (This is the same distinction as in Chapter 6, between weight and intensity.)

The insight-episode. The client says "I've got it!" with elation, and it seems something important has happened. But the experience did not enter the body and stayed on the map. This is the first version from 9.1.

Pseudo-agreement. The client has agreed with the therapist's interpretation — sincerely — but this is agreement with someone else's formulation, not his own lived experience. It changes what the client says, not what he experiences.

What distinguishes a real counter-experience from all three: it engages the body and leaves a lasting trace — an hour later, a day later; it can be named, at least in simple words; it is repeatable, at least in close situations; after it the old configuration has not strengthened; and in it there appears at least a small link to the possibility of action — the experience did not just happen, it opens something that can now be done. The look-alikes usually give one or two signs. A real counter-experience leaves a cumulative trace at once along several lines: in the body, the word, repeatability, action, and the weakening of the old configuration.

9.8. What the therapist does in the moment of counter-experience

When a counter-experience arises, it must be handled very carefully — it is fragile and can roll back within minutes. And almost everything one instinctively wants to do harms it. But first, one caution, without which this whole section can be misread. The therapist does not produce a counter-experience as an object and does not summon it as a technique. He creates the conditions, notices the moment when the new experience begins to happen, and helps it not to fall apart and not to turn back into an explanation. A counter-experience happens; the therapist's role is to prepare the ground and not to get in the way.

One wants to name it, explain it, fix it in words — and too many words close the experience. One wants to generalize: "so now you see that..." — and by this the counter-experience is turned back into an insight, into a map, losing precisely what made it territory. One wants to make a small shift into a large event, to mark it, to rejoice aloud — and by this to inflate what should have stayed small. One wants to move to the next topic while things are going well — and to cut off the moment before it has settled.

What actually works is the reverse. Hold the moment without hurrying it. Name it sparely, or not at all — the experience makes itself, without interpretation. Help it take hold through four channels: let it resonate in the body, sound in the contact, find a word, link to a possible action. And check whether it has a path to repetition — because it is repetition, not the vivid moment in itself, that turns a counter-experience into change.

And one more thing, important for the whole of practice: a counter-experience cannot be the goal of every session. Most of the work is work with conditions: reading the moment, building the sequence, strengthening the field and the capacity. A counter-experience happens on this ground when it is ready. A therapist who makes ICAE the task of every meeting forces it — and forcing closes the very thing he is after.

9.9. The main rule of change

All of this converges into one rule, which stands against the most deeply rooted illusion about therapy — that change comes as a great breakthrough.

> Durable change is not a single breakthrough but an accumulation of minimal integrable counter-experiences, which goes through oscillations, leaves a trace in all four channels, and gradually shifts the reality weight of the old configuration.

From this follows a conclusion that overturns the usual optics. A therapist who looks for big moments — catharsis, breakthrough, the turning-point session — most often misses change, because it goes elsewhere and otherwise. And a therapist who can see and hold small shifts — a two-second glance, one phrase said for the first time, one "nothing happened" — most often helps change to occur and take hold. Change is not loud. It accumulates out of the small, and it can be noticed only once one has stopped waiting for the large.

9.10. Where we go next

With this, the core of the theory of change is assembled. We have everything needed to answer the question with which the book began. Premature rightness (Chapter 1) is the attempt to bring in material, an intervention, or a new possibility before they have become minimally integrable; in the terms of this chapter it often looks like an attempt to summon a counter-experience before it has become minimally integrable. Perpetual stabilization is endless preparation of the ground on which not a single counter-experience is ever allowed to happen. Between them lies all the work: to read the moment (Chapters 5, 6, 7), to build the sequence (Chapter 8), and to let the new experience gain weight through the accumulation of small counter-experiences (this chapter).

Now the next step is needed: to learn to read the very material of experience that all of this works with. What exactly changes in subjective reality when it changes? What forms of time, world, self, salience, affect, the other, action, and meaning do we hear in a session? And how do we keep from turning these forms into types of people, from confusing a configuration with a diagnosis?

This is the subject of the next chapter — phenomenological reading, invariants, and configurations. If Chapters 4–9 gave a grammar of fit, order, and change, Chapter 10 will show what exactly this grammar reads in living clinical material.

Chapter 10. Phenomenological Reading: Invariants and Configurations

10.1. Two clients with one complaint

In a single week two women say almost the same thing to a therapist: "I have no future." The words match down to the intonation. The content of the complaint is identical. And yet these are two different clinical worlds, and they must be worked with differently — and the difference is heard not in the words but in how this "no future" is built in each.

For the first, the future is not absent — it has contracted. She speaks of tomorrow and of next year as though there were no difference between them: everything is close, everything is bearing down, there is no air to breathe. Ask her about plans, and you feel the very space in which a plan might fit narrowing. The future is not empty; it has collapsed toward the almost-present, and no room is left in it for anything to unfold.

For the second it is different. The future as a category is intact in her — she reasons easily about what will happen in a year, builds scenarios, considers options. But not one of these scenarios belongs to her. She describes her future the way a spectator describes someone else's film: in detail, at a distance, without the thread that would tie her to the one who, up ahead, will live it. The future is there — there is no lived "I" that would find itself in it.

The same sentence. But in the first case time is folded; in the second, self-experience. More precisely, in the second case it is not the future itself that is disturbed but the link between the future and the self that could find itself in it. The sequence of work will be different, the dominant constraint most likely lies in different layers, and the minimal counter-experience is different for each. If the therapist hears only the content — "no future"

— he will not see this fork and will work with both the same way. If he hears the form, he will hear that these are two different organizations of experience that have merely coincided in words.

This chapter is about the hearing that allows this to be distinguished. The methodological core is assembled. Now one must learn to hear the very material to which it is applied — the living form of subjective reality as it sounds in the consulting room.

10.2. Why a phenomenological ear is needed after the method

It may seem that after Chapters 4–9 the therapist already has everything. He can read the Cα mode, reality weight, the dominant constraint, build a sequence, notice a counter-experience. What is still missing?

What is missing is an ear for the material itself. All the instruments of the method are instruments for reading the state of the assembly: which mode it is in, with what weight it acts, which layer holds the veto. But they do not say what exactly is assembled right now — what form time, world, self, salience, affect, the other, action, and meaning have taken in this client at this minute. And the method is not applied to a void. It is applied to a concrete form of lived reality, and without hearing that form the instruments hang in the air.

Return to the two women. To determine the dominant constraint in the first, one must first hear that her time is folded — otherwise one will not grasp which layer holds the veto, and over what. To find a minimal counter-experience for the second, one must hear that her link to her own future is torn — otherwise one will offer her a counter-experience to the wrong address. Phenomenological reading comes before the application of the instruments — but before logically, not in time. In a live session the therapist hears form, mode, weight, and veto in one movement; they are to be separated in thought, not in seconds. Logically, though, one must first hear what form of experience is given, and only then ask what can be done with it: reading supplies the instruments with their material. The method answers the question "what to do with this form"; the phenomenological ear answers the prior question "what form this is."

From this comes the formula that holds the whole chapter.

> Phenomenological reading in DDSRF hears not only what the client says but the form of reality within which his words become true.

"No future" is not a lie and not a symptom to be eliminated. Within folded time it is the plain truth: there really is no future where it has collapsed. The therapist who hears the form will stop arguing with the content and begin working with the reality in which the content is true.

10.3. An invariant is not a symptom and not a theme

To speak about form precisely, DDSRF introduces the notion of an invariant. The simplest way to introduce it is through its distinction from two neighboring notions with which it is easily confused.

A symptom says what manifests. Insomnia, intrusive thoughts, loss of energy, attacks of anxiety — these are symptoms. They describe an observable disturbance, and diagnosis rests on them. A symptom is useful, but it is silent about how experience is built from within: two people with the same insomnia may live in entirely different worlds.

A theme says what the client talks about. The relationship with the mother, a divorce, work, guilt toward a child — these are themes. A theme is the content of speech, its subject. It matters, but it too is not about form: one can speak about a mother's leaving out of folded time, out of a shame-bound self, out of a collapse of agency — the theme is one, the organization of experience different.

An invariant says how experience is built. Not what manifests and not what is being talked about, but what form time, world, self, salience, affect, the other, action, or meaning have taken in this experience. "The future is folded to the almost-present" is an invariant. "Being seen is experienced as a threat" is an invariant. "Action does not come from me, it happens to me" is an invariant. An invariant is not the whole organization of subjective reality but a repeatable structural feature of experience: a form of time, world, self, salience, affect, the other, action, or meaning. It is the local form within which symptoms and themes acquire their concrete sound.

The name is not chosen by chance. An invariant is what stays constant while the content changes. In one client shame sounds in the theme of appearance, in another in the theme of work, in a third in the theme of sex. The content differs; the form — "being seen destroys" — is one. This is the invariant: what does not change when the themes change, and so it, and not the theme, is the stable target of the clinical ear.

10.4. Form organizes content

From the distinction between invariant and theme follows a rule worth making explicit, because it changes how the therapist listens.

The same content can carry different form. We have already seen this: "no future" in the two women is one content, two invariants. Add the symmetrical observation, no less important: different content can carry one invariant. A client who cannot finish a project, a client who cannot leave a destroying relationship, and a client who cannot get out of bed are speaking about entirely different things. But beneath all three may lie one invariant — "action does not come from me." The content of the three conversations does not overlap. The form is one.

For practice this means the following. If the therapist listens at the level of content, he begins anew each time: a new theme, new work. If he hears the form, he recognizes beneath different themes a repeating organization of experience — and works with it, not with each of its manifestations separately. The three "I cannot"s from the example above are not three problems but one form in three guises, and a shift in the form will resound in all three.

This continues directly from what we know from Chapter 3: suffering is durable because the configuration reproduces itself. It is precisely the form that is reproduced, not the content. This is why work with content — to persuade, to discuss the theme, to go through a particular case — so often fails to hold: the guise changes, the form remains. Phenomenological reading aims at what is reproduced.

Here too is the first defense against an error to which we will return at the end. To hear the form does not mean to ignore the content. The client's content — his life, his themes, his words — remains what the work proceeds with. Form does not cancel content; it only lets the therapist hear which organization of experience speaks behind these words. A therapist who begins to hear only invariants and stops hearing the person will lose more than he gained.

10.5. Eight groups of invariants: an overview, not a catalog

There are many invariants. In the Method Atlas they are gathered and described separately (Appendix H); there are thirty-three of them, organized for convenience into eight functional groups. In this chapter we do not need the whole catalog — we need an ear for the groups themselves, for the eight directions along which subjective reality can be organized. They are useful to know not in order to attach a label but in order to know where to listen.

The eight groups are eight directions of phenomenological hearing. Temporal invariants are forms of time: whether the future is folded, whether the past intrudes into the present, whether time stands still, whether the link between "then" and "now" is torn. World invariants are forms of world: whether the world is flat, narrowed, has lost depth, or, on the contrary, has become excessively significant in every detail. Self invariants are forms of self-experience: whether the self is intact, whether the "I" is experienced as real, whether the person is present in his own experience or observes it from afar. Salience invariants are forms of what comes forward: what seizes attention, what becomes important against one's will, how salience is distributed among threat, loss, possibility.

Further. Affective invariants are forms of emotional tone: whether affect is available at all, whether it is frozen, whether it is experienced as one's own or as alien, whether there are colors or the world is bleached out. Intersubjective invariants are forms of the other and the field: whether the other is present as alive, experienced as dangerous, as merging, as absent, whether one can be with him and remain oneself. Agentic invariants are forms of action and agency: whether action comes from me, whether "I can" is experienced, or action happens to me, or has collapsed altogether. Noetic invariants are forms of meaning and directedness: whether life has a vector, whether meaning holds, or has collapsed, or, on the contrary, has grown into an unbearable overload where everything matters at once.

Salience and meaning are distinguished here, and they are easily confused. Salience answers the question of what comes forward: what seizes attention, what becomes important in the field of experience against one's will. Meaning answers a different question — what it is directed toward: why it is lived, whether life has a vector. A salience invariant is about what is highlighted right now; a noetic one is about whether directedness holds at all.

The eight groups are not eight boxes into which the client is sorted. They are eight sides from which one can listen in to one and the same assembly. In a real person at a real moment usually not all eight are active but several, and they hold together — that is the subject of the next section. The list is needed precisely so that, on hearing "something is wrong with time" or "the other seems lifeless," the therapist knows these are readable forms and not an elusive impression, and can listen in more precisely.

10.6. Invariants assemble into clusters

In living experience invariants do not come singly. They hold in bundles — several forms that support one another and assemble into a recognizable whole. Such a bundle DDSRF calls a cluster.

Return to the first woman from the start of the chapter. Her future is folded — that is a temporal invariant. But beside it there will almost certainly be several more: the world has narrowed to the bearing-down (a world invariant), action has stalled — "what is the point of planning" (an agentic one), affect has taken on a color of no-way-out (an affective one). These forms are not neighbors by chance. Folded time makes the world cramped; a cramped world drains action of sense; stalled action confirms the no-way-out; the no-way-out folds time still further. The cluster holds itself — by the same recursion we described in Chapter 3.

In a working formulation of a cluster, three to five invariants are most often enough. Fewer, and we are perhaps still seeing a single form, not yet settled into a stable bundle. More, and it is worth checking whether the therapist is trying to describe everything at once instead of singling out the load-bearing bundle, the one that actually holds the assembly right now. This is a rule of formulation, not a law of experience: sometimes reality organizes around one or two vivid invariants, sometimes in complex clinical pictures more are heard — but for a case card it matters to single out the load-bearing ones. It is the cluster, not the single invariant, that fills the field of the active phenomenological cluster in the DDSRF Case Card (Method Atlas, Appendix A): clinically we are interested not in an isolated form but in the group of forms that is organizing the client's reality together right now.

And one more thing, important for all that follows. A cluster belongs to the moment, not to the person. The same woman on another day, in another field, in another Cα mode, may assemble differently: the future will unfold, action will revive. A cluster is a snapshot of the current assembly, not a portrait of the personality. We will now carry this distinction to its end, because it is what separates phenomenological reading from diagnosis.

10.7. Configurations are not diagnoses

When a particular cluster of invariants assembles in a client again and again — not at a single moment but as a stable way in which his reality comes together over and over — we speak of a configuration. A configuration in DDSRF is a stable form of the organization of subjective reality: a recurring cluster that reproduces itself through the cycles of assembly.

The word already sounded in Chapter 3, and here we assemble it in full. A configuration is not a recurring pattern of behavior and not a character trait. It is a pattern of the assembly of experience that confirms itself in each next cycle and therefore holds over time. The shame organization of the self is a configuration: the client assembles reality again and again so that being seen threatens destruction, and each cycle confirms it.

And here is the pivotal distinction of the whole chapter, for whose sake it is being written. A configuration is not a diagnosis. The difference is not cosmetic; it changes everything.

A diagnosis in clinical systems usually serves a different task: it helps describe a disorder, a state, risk, prognosis, communication between specialists, and a possible type of help. A configuration solves another task — it describes how subjective reality is being assembled right now. So a configuration does not answer the question "what disorder does the client have"; it answers the question "what organization of experience is active now and how does it hold itself." This is a mobile characteristic of the moment, not a category of belonging. One cannot "have" a configuration the way one has a diagnosis. A configuration can be active today and inactive tomorrow; within a single session the active configurational organization can change — one giving way to another when the field or the mode shifts. The client does not "be" a shame organization — the shame organization of the self is active in him right now, and that is an entirely different statement.

From this follows the practical point as well. A configuration cannot be treated as a nosological unit — nosology is treated, a form of assembly is read. It is worked with differently: one sees how it assembles experience right now, where it holds the veto, what minimal counter-experience could disrupt its self-confirmation — the one its cycle cannot immediately absorb. To name a configuration is not to attach a label but to grasp what work the assembly is doing right now. It is an instrument of reading, not of classification, and the moment a configuration begins to sound like a type of client, it stops being an instrument of DDSRF and becomes a diagnosis under another name.

10.8. Ten prototypes and five families

There are, in principle, as many configurations as there are stable clusters. But clinical practice runs again and again into a few recurring forms — frequent enough that it is worth giving them names and recognizing them on sight. DDSRF singles out ten prototypical configurations (CCP). They are unfolded in full in the Method Atlas (Appendix I) — with their invariant composition, typical dominant constraint, frequent reading errors; here I only name them, to give a map and not a territory.

Here are the ten. Compression of the future (CCP-1) — the future folded to the almost-present, that very first woman. Intrusion of the past (CCP-2) — the past has not passed, it lasts in the present as something happening now. Defensive clarity (CCP-3) — reality is assembled with a deceptive sharpness in which everything is "clear," and this clarity defends against unbearable uncertainty. Shame organization of the self (CCP-4) — being seen is experienced as a threat of destruction. Attachment without differentiation (CCP-5) — the other is needed to the point of inseparability, and to be oneself beside him is impossible. Collapse of agency (CCP-6) — "I can" has vanished, action does not come from the subject. Action without symbolization (CCP-7) — action is there, but it does not pass through meaning, it discharges before becoming experience. Noetic overload (CCP-8) — there is not too little meaning but unbearably much, everything matters at once. Intersubjective absence (CCP-9) — the other is not present as alive, the field has emptied of people. Frozen transition (CCP-10) — the person is stuck between the old organization and the new, and neither holds.

Ten names are hard to hold in the head at once, so for navigation — and for navigation only — it is convenient to group them into five families. Let me state at once what these families are not, because otherwise they will immediately turn into the very thing the whole chapter warns against. Families are not diagnoses, not new configurations, and not a theoretical level. They are a pedagogical grouping, a way of not getting lost among ten prototypes, and nothing more. They need not be equal in size and make no claim to completeness.

The first family — temporal-transitional configurations: compression of the future, intrusion of the past, frozen transition (CCP-1, 2, 10). What unites them is that time is out of order — the link between “then,” “now,” and “later.” The second — self-protective: defensive clarity and the shame organization of the self (CCP-3, 4). Here the assembly is organized around the defense of the self — from uncertainty or from destroying visibility. The third — intersubjective-attachment: attachment without differentiation and intersubjective absence (CCP-5, 9). Both forms are about how the other is out of order: too much of him to the point of merging, or none of him at all. The fourth — agentic-action: collapse of agency and action without symbolization (CCP-6, 7). Both are about a disorder of action: it is absent, or it is there, bypassing meaning. The fifth — noetic-meaning: noetic overload (CCP-8). In this family there is so far one prototype, and that is fine — a family solves a task of orientation, not of symmetry. Other noetic forms — collapse of meaning, thinning of meaning, loss of directedness — more often appear as invariants within different configurations; in the list of prototypes it is precisely overload that is singled out, because it forms a stable, self-standing configurational logic.

The map is deliberately left a map. Whoever wants the territory — the invariant composition of each prototype, its typical veto, its look-alikes — will find it in the Method Atlas. Here the principle matters more: ten recognizable forms, grouped for convenience into five, are supports for attention, not cells for clients.

10.9. The vertical axis: levels of stability of the assembly, O1–O5

Everything described so far lacks one dimension. Invariants, clusters, and configurations answer the question of which form is assembled right now.

But there is another question, no less clinical: how stably the assembly itself holds under the current load — whether it will stay whole under pressure or begin to fall apart. DDSRF marks this vertical axis as O1–O5.

O1 — stable organization. R(t) is sufficiently coherent; self, time, the other, and action hold; the system can withstand novelty and contradiction without disintegration.

O2 — traumatically fragile organization. Coherence usually holds but drops under certain triggers, affects, or relational loads; outside them the assembly can look stable.

O3 — borderline-unstable organization. The assembly switches rapidly; the other, the field, and the reality weight of experiences sharply change the availability of self and action from session to session and within a session.

O4 — dissociatively fragmented organization. The coherence of self, memory, body, or agency can fall apart into states that hold together poorly.

O5 — psychotically disorganizing organization. The field of shared reality is disturbed; unusual connections, aberrant salience, or disturbances of reality testing begin to organize R(t).

A word at once on how to read this axis, because it is easily misread. O1–O5 is not a diagnosis and not an assessment of the person, but neither is it a neutral "non-scale": it is an axis of integrative stability and the risk of disorganization of the current assembly. It shows not "what kind of person" but how stably the current assembly withstands load — and, like everything in this chapter, it refers to the moment: the same person in different sessions may turn out to be at different levels.

Why this axis matters clinically. It speaks directly of the permissible load — of the very thing with which the whole book began. The less stable the assembly, the lower the permissible integrative load and the more safety, specialized assessment, and supervision count. The same configuration at O1 and at O4 calls for different work: what at a stable level would be a useful counter-experience fragments at a level of disorganization risk. The shame organization of the self in a client with a stable assembly and in a client whose coherence falls apart under load are, in essence, two different clinical situations under one configuration name. The horizontal (which form) and the vertical (how stably it holds) are read together: the first says what you are working with, the second says what load it will withstand right now. A detailed marking of the levels with indicators is in the Method Atlas; for practice what matters most is to read this axis as stability and risk of disorganization, not as a label of severity, and to remember that it too is about the moment.

10.10. To name an invariant is not to understand the person

This whole chapter has given the therapist a vocabulary: invariants, clusters, configurations, prototypes, families, levels of stability. The vocabulary is powerful, and precisely for that reason the chapter must be closed with a warning, without which it is dangerous.

To name an invariant is not to understand the person. To say “here is a shame organization of the self, O2, a cluster of four invariants” is not to understand the person sitting across from you. It is to hear how his reality is built right now — and only that. Between “I hear the form of his experience” and “I understand him” lies the whole person: his history, his words, what no map captures. Phenomenological reading is a way of listening better, not a replacement for listening.

The danger here is real and worth naming directly. A good vocabulary tempts. Having received names for forms, the therapist begins to hear names instead of the person: the client turns into “a CCP-4 at O2,” living speech into material for classification, and the conversation itself imperceptibly becomes a sorting. This is the same error as a diagnostic label, only subtler and more convincing, because it looks not like crude classification but like phenomenological precision — and seems attuned where in fact it closes the ear. The minute an invariant becomes a label, it stops helping one hear and begins to hinder.

So let us gather the defense into one line and hold it. An invariant is not a symptom. A configuration is not a diagnosis. A family is not a type of person. A level of stability is not a diagnosis and not an assessment of personality. All of this is maps for reading how experience is organized, not a classification of personality. A map is needed so as not to get lost; but a person is not a map, and whoever confuses the one with the other will get lost the more surely the more detailed his map.

Phenomenological reading returns us to the formula with which the chapter began: to hear not only what the client says but the form of reality within which his words become true. This form is not he himself. It is what he lives in right now, and to hear it is to gain a chance of helping him live otherwise.

10.11. Where we go next

Now we have both the method (Chapters 4–9) and an ear for the material to which it is applied (this chapter). The therapist can read the state of the assembly and hear its form. But any reading can be carried out wrongly — and the more powerful the instrument, the more serious the error. We have already run into this risk several times: to take a label for understanding, a cluster for a type of person, a level of stability for a label of severity. These errors are not accidental; they have recurring forms, and one can learn to recognize them.

The next chapter is about errors of reading and about how DDSRF is used in supervision: how DDSRF is read wrongly, what distortions are introduced by the therapist's school, his anxiety, his wish for certainty — and why it is precisely the examination of one's own reading errors that makes DDSRF especially useful in supervision. From how the material is built we move to how our own reading of that material is built.

Chapter 11. Errors of Clinical Reading and DDSRF in Supervision

11.1. When precise reading begins to hear instead of the therapist

The therapist listens to the client and hears the form. Everything seems clear: here is a shame organization of the self. The client avoids being seen, apologizes for every expression of herself, expects appraisal in advance, shrinks under the other's gaze. The formulation is precise — perhaps the best the therapist has reached in months of work.

And it is precisely at this moment that the risk begins. Before the formulation the therapist was listening to the client. After the formulation he may begin to listen to his own formulation.

The therapist begins to work with visibility, with shame, with the safety of the field. The work does not move. The client comes in more and more tired, says that at work "it was all terrible again." The therapist hears this as confirmation: she has once more experienced herself as appraised, the shame organization has assembled again. Every session confirms the formulation — and every session passes it by.

In supervision a detail surfaces for which there had been no room in the formulation. The client's boss systematically humiliates employees in public. Her contract is unstable, she is afraid of losing her place, the chance of protecting herself is almost nil. And the supervisor asks: what if it is not only a shame organization here — what if the life-world is right now actually producing humiliation?

And the formulation turns over. The shame remains active; perhaps it really is the client's long-standing configuration. But the dominant constraint right now is not in the shame and not in the field of therapy but in Λ — in the real environment where humiliation continues from day to day. We already saw in Chapter 7 that while the veto is held by the life-world, inner work without a change of conditions is premature — and worse, it begins to sound like a subtle accusation: "you ought to experience differently what is objectively destroying you." For months the therapist had been helping the client bear humiliation better, instead of seeing that the first step had to be not inner processing but protection from the environment that keeps producing that humiliation.

It is worth naming directly what happened here, because this is the subject of the whole chapter. The therapist was not stupid, inexperienced, or inattentive. He did not "apply DDSRF badly." He used one of its layers precisely: he heard the real form. The error was elsewhere — he stopped at this precise form too early and ceased to check what else was holding the situation. An error of clinical reading often begins not where the therapist understood nothing but where he understood too quickly.

This chapter is about such errors. Not in order to frighten the therapist or catch him out, but exactly the reverse. The powerful language that Chapters 4–10 gave helps one hear more precisely — but for that very reason it is also able to begin hearing instead of us. The maturity of the apparatus is not that it spares one from errors but that it makes them visible, nameable, and revisable. Next we will go through eight typical classes of reading error, and then through how DDSRF works in supervision, turning a formulation from a verdict into a hypothesis.

11.2. A reading error is not a moral failure

Before taking apart the classes of error, the extra weight must be lifted off them. A list of errors is easily read as a list of accusations — and then the therapist begins to read the chapter with mounting shame, which by itself makes his reading worse. So let us say it plainly: reading errors are inevitable, and this is not a defect of the therapist but a property of the material itself.

Clinical material is many-layered and is not given all at once. The therapist always works with an incomplete picture and always with hypotheses, otherwise work is impossible: to act, one must settle on something. A hypothesis is not an error. A hypothesis is a working instrument. DDSRF does not promise reading without hypotheses and does not promise hypotheses without misses. It promises something else: a language in which a miss can be noticed and named before it becomes months of work going the wrong way.

From here comes a formula worth holding through the whole chapter. Bad work does not begin where the therapist erred in reading. It begins where the therapist stopped noticing that his reading is a hypothesis. An error of the first kind is corrected at the next session. An error of the second kind can last for years, because the therapist fits each new observation into the already-accepted formulation — as in the vignette above, where the client's fatigue was read as confirmation of the shame rather than as a signal that the formulation is incomplete.

All eight classes of error below are forms of one and the same thing: a hypothesis that has imperceptibly become a certainty. The difference between them is in which reading instrument the transition occurred on — form, mode, weight, veto, order, change, map, or domain. So it is useful to know them separately: knowing the typical place of the slip, one notices the slip earlier.

And through all eight runs one common error, the root one for the whole book — the one named back in Chapter 4: the therapist judges an action by its rightness, not by its fit. "This is the right interpretation," "this is the needed exposure," "this is an important question," "this is the precise name of the configuration" — each of these judgments may be true, and the action will still not land. Reading errors begin where the therapist asks only "is this right" and stops asking: "does this action correspond to the current capacity of the client, the therapist, and the field right now." The eight classes below are eight typical places where rightness substitutes itself for fit.

11.3. The error of content: the therapist hears the theme instead of the form

The most frequent error is the simplest. The client speaks about work, and the therapist works with work. The client speaks about relationships — the therapist works with relationships. The client says "I have no future" — the therapist helps build plans. The reading goes by the content of speech, by what the client is talking about, and does not reach the form — how the experience in which this content becomes true is built.

This is a direct continuation of Chapter 10: a theme is not a form, a symptom is not an invariant. The content suggests the theme but says nothing about which invariant lies beneath it. "No future" may be a compression of time, or a rupture of the self's link to the future; "I can't decide" may be a collapse of agency, or a flatness of a world in which no choice weighs anything. A therapist who works with content begins anew each time; a therapist who hears the form recognizes beneath different themes one organization of experience.

This error is treacherous in that it does not look like an error. The therapist does meaningful, relevant work: the client brought a theme — he works with it, and from the outside everything seems right. The signal of trouble here is not that the work is wrong but that it does not accumulate: theme after theme is taken apart conscientiously, and nothing shifts in the client's experience, because beneath the changing themes one unheard form holds. When work by content goes on for months and does not add up to movement, this is the first reason to ask whether the therapist is hearing themes where he needs to hear the form.

The counter-example holds the whole section. The client says he sees no future, and the therapist conscientiously helps him plan: goals for the year, small steps, a schedule. The plans do not take — not because they are bad but because the very lived space of the future is compressed in the client, and there is nowhere to put a plan. The work is precise by content and off the mark by form. A theme says what the client is talking about. A form says in what reality he is saying it. Until the therapist has heard the reality, his precise actions on the theme will not land.

11.4. The error of mode: the therapist misreads $C\alpha$

The second error is in reading the mode of the assembly. A reminder from Chapter 5: the mode is determined not by the content of the experience but by what the system does with novelty, and there are five modes — fragmenting, defensively closed, stabilizing, exploratory, transitional. To confuse them is to bring in an intervention the current mode cannot take.

The main pair, as in Chapter 5, is the defensively closed and the stabilizing: alike on the outside, opposite in essence. Take defensive closure for stabilization, and the therapist endlessly "reinforces" what is in fact a closing-down, helping the old reality hold. Take stabilization for closure, and the therapist starts bringing in load where the system is only just gathering coherence, and brings it down. There are other substitutions too: the exploratory mode is taken for an integration already accomplished, and one celebrates a change that is not yet there; the transitional mode for a stable result, and support is withdrawn too early; the fragmenting for "strong affect," and one deepens what is in fact a disintegration of coherence, not a breakthrough.

The root of all these substitutions is one: the mode was read by the client's words, not by the fate of novelty. The client speaks with conviction — the therapist hears stability; the client weeps — the therapist hears a breakthrough; the client agrees — the therapist hears openness. But conviction, tears, and agreement by themselves say nothing yet about what the system did with the new. The error of mode is an error in reading what the system does with novelty. It is checked not by intonation but by what remained afterward: did the new land, was it turned into a confirmation of the old, or did it destroy coherence.

11.5. The error of weight: an experience taken for a thought

The third error is in reading reality weight. From Chapter 6: weight RW0–RW4 says how far an experience organizes the client's life in spite of his rational agreement, and work with RW2 differs fundamentally from work with RW4. The error here is to treat a high weight as though it were low; a particular case of it is to work with RW3 as though it were RW1.

The scenario is typical and deceptive. The client understands, formulates, agrees: "yes, I know I am not to blame," "yes, with my reason I understand that I am loved." The therapist hears rational agreement and decides one can work through content — bring arguments, look for proof, persuade. But the experience has a high weight: it acts as world, not as thought, and governs the body, expectations, and actions independently of what the client says about it. Arguments against RW3 do not land — they bounce off or generate pseudo-agreement, agreement with the formulation without a shift in the experience. From here too the close error: to take that very agreement for a drop in weight and move on, leaving the reality untouched. And separately — to fail to see RW4 and the boundary of safety: in a self-sealed reality a head-on refutation is not merely useless, it raises the risk of closing-down.

The symmetrical error exists too, though it occurs more rarely: to conduct deep, many-layered work where the weight is in fact low and a simple reframing would have sufficed. But clinically the first is more dangerous. The error of weight is to work with an experience as with a thought when it acts as reality. To argue with what weighs as world is like proving to a person that the floor beneath him is not real: the argument is correct, and he goes on standing on the floor.

11.6. The error of veto: the therapist works with the active rather than the blocking

The fourth error is in reading the dominant constraint. From Chapter 7: a layer can be active (takes part in the assembly), load-bearing (substantially holds the configuration), and with veto power (blocks the next step), and one must work with what holds the veto, not with what is more noticeable. The error of veto is to follow the visible.

And the visible and the blocking often do not coincide. Shame is active and sounds in every phrase — but the veto is held by the field, and while contact is unsafe, work with shame does not land. Anxiety is noticeable — but the veto is at the body, and without bodily regulation talking about the anxiety only winds it up. Helplessness is obvious — but the veto is at the life-world, as in the opening vignette, and no inner work will shift what continues to destroy from outside. The narrative is vivid and detailed — but the veto is at the coherence thresholds, and deepening the narrative leads to fragmentation. In every case the therapist works with what asks for attention by itself, bypassing what silently holds the door shut.

It is important that the veto hypothesis itself is not an error; the error is in not testing it. Chapter 7 gave three tests for this: the failure test (which interventions have already stopped landing), the small-support test (which small shift immediately raises coherence), and the counterfactual test (if this layer were temporarily stabilized, would the next step become possible).

And the rule of triangulation: a veto hypothesis is strong only when at least two independent sources point to one layer. The therapist in the vignette ran not a single test — otherwise the failure test would have shown at once that work with shame has not landed for months, and that is the first sign that the veto is not where he is looking for it. The error of veto is to work with what is visible, bypassing what makes the next step impossible.

11.7. The error of order: a right action out of its place

The fifth error is in time. From Chapter 8: an intervention has not only content but also a place in the sequence, and a right step taken out of its place stops being right. Two forms of this error are symmetrical.

The first is too early: premature rightness, the central problem of the whole book. The therapist sees the goal and goes to it in a straight line, bypassing what should have become possible earlier. He names the trauma while the coherence threshold is too low; demands action while agency is not assembled; leads toward meaning while a bodily veto holds. The step is right — but before its place, and so it gives closing-down, fragmentation, or pseudo-agreement instead of change.

The second is never: perpetual stabilization. The therapist is so afraid of overloading that he endlessly regulates, supports, and holds safety, but never creates the conditions for a counter-experience. The system is intact and does not change. Here one should hold the caution from Chapter 8: there are cases — severe trauma, deep dysregulation, crisis — where stabilization is the work, and the stabilizing mode in Chapter 5 is described as a full-fledged one, not an insufficient one. The error is not in stabilization itself but in its having become permanent and taken the place of change.

These two forms feel different in the room, and this helps catch them. Premature rightness is often accompanied by closing-down, fragmentation, pseudo-agreement, or rollback — the system replies that the step is early. Perpetual stabilization feels deceptively good: the sessions are warm, the alliance strong, the client feels supported — and that is precisely why it is harder to notice, since nothing outwardly points to trouble except that time passes and no new availabilities of life appear. The first is given away by the system's reaction, the second by its absence. Both forms are the loss of one question. The error of order is the loss of the question: what must become possible earlier?

11.8. The error of change: an event in the room taken for a change in life

The sixth error is in reading change itself. From Chapter 9: insight changes the map, counter-experience changes the availability of the territory, and a real counter-experience has convincing look-alikes. The error here is to take a look-alike for change.

Chapter 9 described several look-alikes of counter-experience, and each tempts in its own way; here one more, separate error is added to them — to take a single counter-experience for an already-consolidated change. The client said "I've got it!" — an insight-episode, the elation is there, but the experience stayed on the map and did not enter the body; the therapist thinks something has changed. The client wept, the session was powerful — catharsis, the affect roared through and left no trace; the therapist thinks a shift has occurred. The client agreed with the formulation — verbal agreement without a change of weight: what he says changed, not what he experiences; the therapist thinks an ICAE has arisen. And the fourth form, the added one: a counter-experience happened once — and the therapist considers that structural change has taken hold, forgetting that change is non-linear, goes through oscillations, and holds not on one vivid moment but on repetition.

Behind all four is one substitution: the vividness of an event in the room is taken for a change in the availability of life. But, as was said back in Chapter 6, the force of affect does not equal weight: a storm may roar through without shifting anything, while a quiet "I said it and was not rejected" may shift it. A real counter-experience is recognized not by vividness but by a cumulative trace — in the body, in the word, in repeatability, in the link to action, in the fact that the old configuration has not become more convincing and sealed after it.

There is a price to this error worth naming. Having taken a look-alike for change, the therapist withdraws support, closes the theme, moves on — and the ground is not ready, and the client rolls back. A rollback by itself is not a failure: change is non-linear. The failure is that the therapist did not expect it, because he considered the change already accomplished — and now reads the rollback as regression or resistance, when in fact he simply overestimated what happened. So one reading error drags another along with it: an unread look-alike turns into a misunderstood rollback. The error of change is to take an event in the room for a change in the availability of life.

11.9. The error of the map: an invariant, CCP, or O-level becomes a label

The seventh error is a direct continuation of Chapter 10 and, in a sense, the main danger of the whole apparatus. The vocabulary the book gave the therapist — invariant, cluster, configuration, CCP, family, O-level — can help one hear, or can begin to hear instead of him. The boundary is thin and runs exactly where the name of a form stops opening attention and begins to close it.

The symptom is recognizable. “This is a CCP-4.” “He is O3.” “She has intersubjective absence.” “This is defensive clarity.” It is said — and the therapist stops listening, because it seems to him that he already knows. The code that in Chapter 10 was a support for attention turns into a cell, and the living person is folded into it. This is the same error as a diagnostic label, only subtler: it looks like phenomenological precision and so seems not classification but depth — as in the opening vignette, where “shame organization” was correct and yet closed the therapist’s ear.

The defense against this error is not a refusal of the vocabulary but a check on how it acts. The code is for attention, not for power over the case. And there is a simple sign by which the living use is told from the dead. A named form should make the therapist more curious, not more certain. If, on hearing “shame organization,” the therapist begins to ask more finely — by what exactly this shame holds now, what supports it, where the veto is — the map is working. If he settles at this and stops asking, the map has become a label, and it is time to return to the person.

It is worth noting that it is not the novice who is more prone to this error but the one who has mastered the language well. The more confidently the therapist commands the vocabulary, the faster a formulation assembles for him and the more convincing it sounds — to himself first of all. Fluency in DDSRF, like any clinical fluency, carries its own risk: it speeds recognition, and recognition is so easily taken for understanding. So the sign of curiosity here is not a polite recommendation but a working safeguard: it tells the one who uses the map from the one whom the map has begun to use.

11.10. The error of domain, field, and conditions: the therapist reads too narrowly

The eighth error is the broadest; it unites several slips into one class: the therapist reads the field of causality too narrowly and goes blind to part of what holds the experience. From Chapter 3 these are P-reduction and M-reduction, but adjoining them are the omission of Λ, the omission of S(t), and the invisibility of the therapist himself in the field.

P-reduction — work only with the experience while ignoring the conditions. The therapist hears the subtle phenomenology but does not see the insomnia, the medication, an untreated somatic condition, a dangerous environment. A client with hypothyroidism gets existential work on the meaning of fatigue; a client in a genuinely threatening situation hears that his fear is a distorted perception. M-reduction is the reverse: the therapist explains everything by the body, trauma, neurobiology, attachment, and loses the form of the experience, reducing a living experience to its mechanism. Both are equally blind, simply in different directions.

Here too belong the omission of the life-world Λ (the whole opening vignette is built on it: an inner problem where the environment produces humiliation) and the omission of the intersubjective field. The latter is worth naming separately, because it is the easiest to miss: the therapist sees the client but does not see himself as part of S(t) — does not notice the counterload, the way his own anxiety, fatigue, or need for a result enters the assembly and distorts the reading. The client's reality is assembled not before the therapist but together with him, and a therapist who has dropped out of his own field of vision reads only half.

It is important that no domain is privileged — the error is symmetrical. A mechanistic explanation may be entirely plausible and still clinically premature if it substitutes for the experience. A phenomenological description may be subtle and precise and still clinically incomplete if it does not see the conditions that hold this experience. DDSRF gives preference neither to form nor to conditions: it requires holding both languages at once and remembering that blindness to either makes the work incomplete, and sometimes premature. The error of domain is precise reading in one language that has gone blind to the other.

11.11. DDSRF in supervision: how to make reading revisable

The eight classes of error are united by one thing: a hypothesis that has stopped being felt as a hypothesis. So the antidote is one too — to return to a formulation the status of the revisable. This is the main work of DDSRF in supervision. DDSRF in supervision is needed not to prove a formulation right but to make it revisable.

This must be said against the natural course of supervision. Bringing a case, the therapist usually wants his reading confirmed: he has already invested in the formulation and is seeking agreement. Supervision that limits itself to confirming the formulation entrenches exactly the certainty out of which the errors of this chapter grow. Supervision in the language of DDSRF does the reverse — it does not assess whether the formulation is right but asks what it rests on and where it might have slipped. The tone here decides everything: not "here is where the therapist erred" but "live reading inevitably slips somewhere; let us look where." Without shame, without catching out misses, without condescension — otherwise the therapist will begin to defend the formulation instead of revising it.

In practice this is a set of questions that pass through all the instruments of the book — not a protocol but a direction of looking. What did the therapist hear first — the theme, the symptom, the invariant, or his own theory? In what Cα mode was the assembly at the moment of the key intervention? What reality weight did the experience he worked with carry? What at that moment was active, what load-bearing, and what held the veto — and was this checked by tests? What was done prematurely, and what should have become possible earlier? Was it a counter-experience or one of its look-alikes? What was happening with the therapist himself — what counter-load did he carry, how did he enter S(t)? And has some DDSRF notion become a label on which the reading stopped?

Each of these questions corresponds to one of the eight errors — this is the way to catch them in one's own work. But the point of supervision is not to check the therapist against a list of eight misses. The point is to return mobility to the formulation: to show that it was a good hypothesis, and for that very reason worth testing, not guarding. In this lies the whole turn the book proposes for mature clinical thinking. If Chapter 10 gave the therapist an ear for the form of the client's experience, this chapter gave an ear for one's own reading — the ability to hear what one is hearing and to ask whether one believed it too soon. Good supervision in DDSRF does not make the therapist less confident. It makes his confidence testable.

11.12. Where we go next

By this point the book has given the method, an ear for the material, and an ear for one's own reading of that material. One last question remains, without which the apparatus cannot count as mature: what are its boundaries. With which schools is DDSRF compatible and where the line of that compatibility runs; what in DDSRF is testable and what remains a clinical heuristic or an open question; where it works and where it is more honest to say it does not apply.

The next, concluding chapter is about compatibility, boundaries, and testability. A strong theory is recognized not only by what it can do but by how clearly it knows what it cannot. From reading our own errors we move to reading the boundaries of the apparatus itself.

Chapter 12. Compatibility, Boundaries, and Testability

12.1. Why a strong theory needs boundaries

The stronger the language, the greater the temptation to apply it everywhere. By this chapter DDSRF has already given a great deal: a language of subjective reality and its assembly, of integrability and fit, of Cα modes, reality weight, the dominant constraint, sequence, counter-experience, phenomenological invariants, and, finally, the errors of one's own reading. This is a coherent apparatus, and coherence is in itself persuasive — so much so that one wants to apply it to anything at all and to hear in it an answer to any clinical question. It is precisely here, at the peak of persuasiveness, that the apparatus passes its main test of maturity.

This chapter is about three things, without which the apparatus would remain a temptation rather than an instrument. Where DDSRF is compatible with other approaches and how it translates into their language. Where its boundaries run — clinical and ethical — and where it is obliged to stay silent. And which of its statements are already knowledge and which are still hypotheses, and how they can be tested. This is a chapter not about the expansion of the apparatus but about its discipline.

Its logic is the reverse of what a strong theory is pulled toward. The natural movement of any school is to expand, to explain more and more, to draw neighboring fields into its vocabulary. DDSRF moves the other way: it outlines what it does not do, before whom it gives way, what it has not yet proven. This is not weakness and not caveats out of politeness. A strong theory is recognized not by explaining everything but by knowing the boundaries of its own applicability. We ended Chapter 11 with the thought that maturity lies in revisability; this chapter carries it to its end, applying that same revisability to the apparatus itself.

The cost of not observing the boundaries is not abstract. An apparatus applied indiscriminately begins to sound like an explanation where what was needed was a halt: suicidal risk is redescribed as a “drop in integrative capacity,” a destructive environment as a “configuration requiring integration,” a somatic cause of a state as a “bodily veto,” and behind an elegant formulation the necessary action vanishes. The more persuasive the language, the more plausible such a redescription sounds — and the more dangerous it is. So the boundaries in this chapter are not an appendix to the apparatus but a part of it: without them a strong language becomes a way of not seeing what is most important to see.

12.2. DDSRF is not a school of therapy

This must be said plainly and early, because everything else in the chapter depends on it. DDSRF has no techniques of its own. It does not replace psychoanalysis, CBT, ACT, DBT, CFT, EMDR, somatic, systemic, existential, or humanistic approaches, and does not stand in a row with them as one more method among methods. It does not tell the therapist what exactly to do in the room — to interpret, to set up an experiment, to work with the body, to seek values. Techniques remain with the schools the therapist takes them from.

DDSRF works at a different level. It does not answer the question “which technique to use”; it answers the question “can this technique land now.” The psychoanalyst decides what counts as a correct interpretation; the CBT or process-based therapist, what counts as a successful behavioral experiment, a cognitive shift, or a change of process; the systemic therapist, what counts as a fitting systemic intervention. Into these criteria of rightness DDSRF does not intervene. It only adds to the question of rightness the question of fit — whether this right action will land in the current assembly or turn out to be premature.

From this comes the precise formulation of its own role. To say “I work by the DDSRF method” would be inaccurate: there is no method as a set of techniques. More precise is something else: “I use DDSRF as a grammar of case formulation, sequence, and integrability within my own clinical school.” A grammar does not compete with the words of a language — it sets how words connect into meaningful speech. So here too: if, after this book, a CBT therapist comes to understand more precisely when his method lands and when it is premature, this is a success of DDSRF; if he abandons CBT for the sake of DDSRF, this is its failure.

What this gives in practice is seen in how the therapist's vision changes without changing his school. The psychoanalyst remains a psychoanalyst but sees more precisely: when an interpretation lands in an open mode and when it meets defensive closure; where the client's veto power lies; what "an interpretation is premature here" means not in a general analytic but in an operational sense. The CBT therapist remains a CBT therapist but distinguishes when a behavioral experiment rests on a sufficient weight of the alternative and when it runs into a self-sealed reality into which a refutation does not land — and then "low motivation" turns out to be not a defect of the client but a sign of unreadiness for this load right now. The school stays the same; what becomes more precise is the reading of the moment in which it works.

12.3. The compatibility matrix: how DDSRF translates into the language of the schools

Compatibility is best seen in translation. Below are not an encyclopedia of schools and not an analysis of their theories, but short bridges: in what language a school describes the moment, what this translates into in the language of DDSRF, and what DDSRF does not assert in doing so. The full matrix is gathered in the Method Atlas, Appendix J; it does not replace the literature of these schools and does not retell their theory — its task is to show how the language of DDSRF can be translated into already-existing clinical languages. Here, only the principle. And the tone everywhere is one: not "DDSRF explains your school," but "DDSRF is translatable into your language."

Begin with the psychodynamic and relational languages. In psychoanalysis there work transference, interpretation, containment, the unconscious, the choice of the moment. In the language of DDSRF this is the field of the other S(t), the Cα mode, the dominant constraint, and sequence; "premature interpretation" acquires an operational sense — an intervention into a defensively closed mode. DDSRF, in doing so, replaces neither transference nor work with the unconscious, history, and deep symbolization.

Next, the process and behavioral languages. In CBT and process-based CBT there work beliefs, schemas, exposure, behavioral experiments, processes of change; translation goes through reality weight, predictive activity $P\sigma$, load and capacity, the minimal counter-experience. DDSRF does not say that cognitive work is superficial — it says that a cognitive change must become integrable. In ACT — defusion, acceptance, values, psychological flexibility; translation through reality weight, noetic invariants, and counter-experience. DDSRF does not replace the flexibility model but specifies which layer holds the fusion at a given moment.

Adjoining the process languages are the skills-based ones. In DBT there work regulation, skills, dialectics, crisis safety; translation through the bodily base B(t), the thresholds Θ, the $C\alpha$ modes, and stabilization as a building-up of capacity; DDSRF does not replace skills training and crisis work. In CFT — shame, self-criticism, threat, soothing, compassion; translation through the reality weight of shame, the field S(t), threat prediction, the minimal counter-experience of safe visibility; DDSRF does not reduce compassion to a technique for lowering shame.

Finally, the bodily, traumatic, systemic, and existential languages. In EMDR and trauma therapy there work the window of tolerance, processing, titration, dual attention, traumatic memory; translation through the thresholds Θ, the body B(t), reality weight, developmental calibration D_cal, and sequence; DDSRF does not replace specialized trauma therapy. In somatic approaches — the body, autonomic regulation, interoception, grounding; translation through B(t), Θ, and the bundle of load, capacity, and field; DDSRF does not assert that the body explains everything. In systemic therapy — relationships, circularity, the family system, patterns of interaction; translation through S(t), the life-world Λ, the field, and the recursivity of assembly from R(t) to R(t+1); DDSRF does not reduce the system to the individual psyche. In existential and humanistic therapy — meaning, freedom, presence, authenticity, encounter; translation through noetic invariants, S(t), and the reality weight of meaning; DDSRF does not dictate the content of meaning and does not substitute a grammar for the living encounter. And in Gestalt and relational approaches the language of contact, boundary, field, and "here-and-now" experiencing can be translated into the language of DDSRF through S(t), the $C\alpha$ mode, the integrative capacity of the field, and the minimal counter-experience; DDSRF, in doing so, does not substitute a grammar for the living work of contact.

Through all the bridges runs one thing. Each school remains itself, with its own techniques and its own criteria of rightness. DDSRF adds a common language for the layer where the schools usually diverge — for the reading of the moment: what is assembled now, which mode, which weight, what holds the veto, what must become possible earlier. This is what makes it translatable rather than competing.

12.4. Boundaries of application

There are states in which DDSRF should not be a self-standing frame. This must be said hard, because a soft formulation here is more dangerous than a sharp one. Suicidal risk; psychotic disorganization; mania and severe affective episodes; severe dissociation; eating disorders with medical risk; active violence; high-risk addictions; somatic and pharmacological causes of a state; legal, social, and safety-related threats — in all these cases what works first is not a reading of the moment but safety, risk assessment, and appropriate specialized help.

This is the same boundary the book already drew in Chapters 2 and 7, and here formulates definitively. Questions of safety stand above any logic of fit and veto. Suicidal risk, violence, psychotic disorganization, medical danger — these are not candidates for a "dominant constraint" with which other layers of the assembly compete. This is a clinical priority that sets the boundary of the work and temporarily suspends the ordinary practice of reading the moment. Where life is at stake, what operates is not the logic of the veto but responsibility for life and the appropriate help.

It matters to say this precisely, for the following reason. DDSRF can indeed help to read the organization of experience in these states too — the stability axis O1–O5, for example, directly describes the zone of disorganization. But to read is not to lead. DDSRF can help one see how experience is built in these states, but it does not replace specialized assessment, crisis work, psychiatry, medicine, legal or social help. The book is written above all for the zone where there is suffering, fragility, and complexity, but the conditions of psychotherapeutic work are preserved: basic safety, sufficient coherence, and the possibility of a supervisable clinical process. In this zone the apparatus works. Beyond it, it remains a language of description but not a guide to action, and to confuse the two is a serious error, not a subtlety.

The difference between “to read” and “to lead” here is not philosophical but practical. A therapist who has noticed along the O5 axis that the client’s reality testing is collapsing has read something correct — and precisely for that reason his next step is not “work with the configuration” but a psychiatric referral. A reading that does not pass into specialized help where it is needed turns from a valuable observation into a dangerous delay. The use of the apparatus in these zones lies exactly in recognizing earlier that one is at a boundary — and, having recognized it, handing the lead to whoever’s field it is.

12.5. Ethical boundaries: integration does not equal adaptation

One boundary must be drawn separately, because it concerns the most central notion of the book: it runs not outside the apparatus but inside its core. Integrability is easily read as a demand: since the talk is of what should “land,” there arises the temptation to hear in this that the client must accept something. This reading is wrong and dangerous, and it must be closed directly.

Integration is not a justification. The integration of trauma does not mean reconciliation with violence. The integration of anger does not mean its suppression. The integration of the reality of a destructive environment does not mean adaptation to it. The opening vignette of Chapter 11 was about exactly this: where the life-world Λ actually produces humiliation, the task is not to help the client bear it better but to name the condition as real and to seek protection, a boundary, a way out, or external help. DDSRF must not become a language in which a client is told “you need to integrate this” where it is more honest to say “this is destroying you, and the work right now is protection.”

The distinction here is precise and worth holding. Integrability answers the question “can this land now,” not the question “should the client accept it.” The first question is descriptive, about the state of the assembly; it carries no “should” within it. The apparatus describes what the current reality is able to take in without closing-down, fragmentation, or pseudo-agreement — and only that. What is worth taking in, what is worth resisting, what is worth defending against and leaving — that is a question of values and safety, not of the throughput of the assembly. DDSRF does not answer it and must not pretend to answer it.

One must be especially careful here with what looks like resistance to integration but is in fact a healthy defense. A client who does not "work through" a relationship with a person who continues to do harm may be not closed but right; an unwillingness to "let go" of anger at a real abuser may be not stuckness but soundness. An apparatus that has forgotten its own descriptiveness risks reading such a defense as an unfitness for integration and beginning to dismantle it gently — and this is perhaps the most serious abuse of the language of DDSRF, because it dresses itself as care. Before asking whether something can land, one sometimes needs to ask whether it should land at all — and that is no longer a question of the apparatus.

12.6. Epistemic status: how knowledge differs from a hypothesis

The maturity of a theory is seen also in how it relates to its own statements. They are not equal in force: something in DDSRF is a working notation, something an observation, something a still-unproven hypothesis. To mix them and present them with the same confidence is to mislead the reader. So that this does not happen, every statement has an epistemic status, a scale ES0–ES5; it is gathered in full in Appendix K, here — its sense.

From the bottom up it looks like this. ES0 — a conceptual frame: the notation R(t), the operator Cα as notation, a way of speaking and not a proven mechanism. ES1 — a phenomenological observation: invariants as descriptive structures of experience, distinguishable in the material; the degree of maturity of a particular invariant may, at that, differ. ES2 — a clinical heuristic: the dominant constraint, the Cα modes — working distinctions, useful at the bedside but not proven as entities. ES3 — a mechanistic hypothesis: M-descriptions, links with the body, prediction, memory — plausible but requiring testing. ES4 — a testable hypothesis: ICAE, the principle of sequence, inter-rater agreement, predictive usefulness — what can and should be put to an empirical test. ES5 — a confirmed statement: and here it must be said honestly that in the current version DDSRF's own new constructs should almost never claim this status. Part of the background clinical and scientific premises it rests on may have high external support, but precisely the DDSRF-specific statements must for now remain more cautious.

The sense of the scale is not self-diminishment. To call R(t) a notation and not a discovery is not to weaken the theory; it is to keep it from passing off a convenient notation as a proven fact. The maturity of DDSRF lies not in asserting everything with the same confidence but in knowing the force of each of its own statements. A reader who sees the status of each notion can lean on the strong and test the weak — and that is more reliable than an even confidence under which it is not visible where knowledge is and where guesswork.

The scale guards against a characteristic failure of young theories — against what may be called inflation of status. A successful notation like R(t) = Cα[…] looks like a formula, and from this it begins to seem as though a measured quantity stands behind it; a beautiful metaphor of the assembly operator imperceptibly begins to sound like a mechanism discovered in the brain. So notation passes itself off as knowledge, and the theory, without noticing it itself, promises more than it has. An explicit status puts on each notion a mark of its real force and thereby keeps the theory's promises within what it can actually present. This is especially important for a two-domain apparatus: M-descriptions, links with the body and prediction, sound temptingly like hard science, and it is they that are most often threatened with an overstatement of status.

12.7. Normative status: where a clinical obligation arises

Epistemic status must be separated from another with which it is easily merged: how far a statement is knowledge — and how far it is a prescription. These are different axes. A theoretical proposition may be no more than a notation and carry no "do this"; a clinical requirement may be obligatory without being a proven mechanism. For this second axis there is its own scale — normative status NS0–NS3.

Briefly: NS0 — no prescription, a purely descriptive proposition. NS1 — clinical caution, a reason to be more attentive. NS2 — a strong recommendation, to depart from which is worth doing only with a clear ground. NS3 — a boundary of safety: a situation where specialized help is required and where the ordinary logic of the apparatus steps back. The two axes diverge clearly in examples. The notation R(t) is ES0 and at the same time NS0: a way of speaking, prescribing nothing. “Do not force traumatic material under falling coherence” is a heuristic moving toward testability (around ES2–ES4), but in normative force it is NS2, a strong recommendation. And “suicidal risk requires a safety assessment” is NS3 independently of any epistemic status: the obligation here does not wait for theoretical proof.

This distinction is mature and practically important. Not every theoretical statement is a clinical prescription, and not every clinical prescription is a proven mechanism. Confusion of the two axes generates two typical errors: to turn a beautiful theoretical notation into an obligatory rule — or, conversely, to postpone a necessary action until the mechanism is proven. Safety does not wait for proofs; notation does not dictate behavior. To hold these axes apart is part of the same discipline as the whole chapter.

To read a statement along both axes at once is a useful habit, and it quickly becomes automatic. “Reality weight is held by several layers” — along the epistemic axis this is so far a heuristic, along the normative one it prescribes nothing concrete: ES2, NS0. “At high RW one contradicting experience is usually not enough unless it passes through the body, the field, the narrative, and action” — the same heuristic support, but already with the normative force of a recommendation: roughly ES2, NS2. “At signs of psychotic disorganization a psychiatric assessment is needed” — along the normative axis this is the boundary of safety NS3, and its force does not depend on what epistemic status the O1–O5 axis itself stands at. One sentence, two independent coordinates — and each answers its own question: how far we know this and how far it obliges.

12.8. How DDSRF can be tested

The question of testability cannot be settled by either boasting or postponement. It is wrong to say that DDSRF is already proven; it is also wrong to wave it off, that testing is needed “someday.” The honest answer is different: which validation exactly corresponds to the nature of this theory. And its nature is two-domain and processual — it describes both the form of experience and its conditions, and the dynamics of their change over time — so there can be no single gold standard here. Testing must go along several converging lines.

The first — phenomenological validation: can invariants and clusters be independently recognized in real material? Methods — qualitative coding, the micro-phenomenological interview, inter-rater agreement. The second — process validation: can one observe in session recordings the transitions of Cα modes, changes in reality weight, the work of the veto, the appearance of counter-experience? Methods — session analysis, conversation analysis, process coding. The third — pragmatic validation: does DDSRF help clinicians formulate a case and choose a sequence better? Methods — training with before-and-after measurement, supervision studies, assessment of the quality of case formulation. The fourth — case series and N=1: documented cases in which sequence, veto, change of weight, and the accumulation of minimal counter-experiences are traced. The fifth — cross-school translatability: can specialists of different schools use DDSRF without losing their own school? Methods — Delphi procedures, cross-school supervisions, expert groups.

The first realistic test could be quite simple. Give several clinicians the same session fragments and see how consistently they distinguish the Cα mode, the level of reality weight, and the presumed dominant constraint. If there is no consistency, the language needs refining until it becomes distinguishable. If it appears after a short training, one can take the next step — to check whether this improves the quality of case formulation and of the supervisory decision. So an abstract program of validation begins with one feasible study, not with a promise to "test it someday."

None of these lines on its own will confirm or refute the theory. Phenomenological recognition without process data will remain description; process correlates without pragmatic use, a laboratory fact without clinical weight. The strength of proof here lies in convergence. DDSRF should be tested not by a single gold standard but by a convergence of methods corresponding to its two-domain and processual nature. This is slower and more modest than one decisive trial, but more honest toward what the theory actually asserts.

It is worth saying plainly what place the familiar gold standard — randomized outcome comparison — occupies. It can be useful for particular applications: for testing DDSRF-based training or the quality of case formulation. But it cannot be the sole and first judge of the theory itself, because DDSRF is not a treatment protocol: it has no techniques of its own whose outcomes could be compared with a control; it is a grammar built into the work of different schools. To ask "does DDSRF, as a self-standing protocol, treat better than a control" is a category error, like testing by a controlled trial the usefulness of grammar for writing. The fitting question is different: does this language help clinicians see the moment more precisely, agree on formulations more reliably, notice prematureness earlier — and is what it describes recognized by independent observers? Such questions are answered not by one trial but by a converging series of different tests, and to demand otherwise is to measure the theory by an instrument not of its nature.

12.9. Where the theory should grow next

From testability follows directly the direction of growth — and it is not toward explaining more. The temptation of a strong theory is to expand: to add new axes, new configurations, new applications, until the language covers everything. This is the path to bloat, not to maturity. DDSRF should grow inward, not outward: testing more precisely the notions it already uses.

The nearest tasks are made of exactly this. To develop a short version of the DDSRF Case Card. To check the inter-rater agreement of invariant recognition — whether two clinicians diverge in reading the same material. To check the reliability of recognizing the levels of reality weight RW0–RW4 as a qualitative clinical instrument. To investigate how reliably the Cα modes are recognized. To gather clinical series that test the principle of sequence. To operationalize ICAE — to specify by what signs a counter-experience differs from its look-alikes not only in words. To test cross-school translatability in practice. To develop a format of training and supervision in which the language is transmitted without distortion.

Behind this list lies one stance with which it is worth ending the conversation about development. A theory becomes stronger not when it expands but when it tests its favorite notions more precisely. The ideas dearest to the author — the assembly operator, counter-experience, the dominant constraint — are the first candidates for rigorous testing, not for protection from it. A readiness to put one's own central notions at risk is the same quality that in Chapter 11 was an ear for one's own errors, only turned now upon the apparatus itself.

It is worth naming the opposite movement too, in order to recognize it. Growth outward looks tempting: to add an axis for one more field of experience, a configuration for digital addiction, a section for couples, for groups, for organizations — and the language seems to become more powerful. In fact, every such expansion that has not passed testing dilutes the apparatus: coverage grows, testability falls, and the theory imperceptibly turns into a worldview that explains everything and risks nothing. The mature path is duller and more honest — to take the notions already at hand and ask of each whether it can be independently recognized, operationalized, tested, or refuted. The book prefers a narrow and testable theory to a broad and persuasive one.

12.10. How this book ends

The book began with one clinical scene: the therapist does an action right in content, and it does not land. Out of that scene grew everything else — the language of subjective reality and its assembly, of integrability and fit, of modes, weight, veto, sequence, counter-experience, phenomenological invariants, and reading errors. The apparatus has turned out large. But its sense lies not in itself.

None of this replaces clinical aliveness, and none of it stands in the place of the meeting of two people in the room. The language of DDSRF is needed not for confidence but for a more precise, more modest, and revisable action. It helps to notice what otherwise slips away: what is assembled now in the client's experience, what does not land and why, what has veto power, what must become possible earlier, and where the therapist's own formulation is asking for revision. It is an instrument of attention, not of power over the case — exactly in the sense Chapter 11 spoke of.

The book did not ask the therapist to change schools, to master a new protocol, or to believe in a new system. It asked for something small and difficult — to hold in mind one question beside the question of rightness: not "is this right," but "can this land now." Everything else — modes, weight, veto, sequence, counter-experience, invariants, reading errors, the statuses of statements — is the unfolding of this one question into a working language. If the reader keeps from the book above all this question, he keeps its main thing.

And so the book's promise too is modest. DDSRF does not promise the therapist an errorless reading. It promises something else: a language in which one can more precisely notice what is assembled now, what does not land, what has veto power, what must become possible earlier, and where the formulation itself requires revision. If, after this book, the therapist becomes not more confident but more precise; not faster but more attentive to order; not more attached to his school or to DDSRF itself, but more able to translate between languages — the book has done its task.

A strong clinical theory does not replace the encounter. It helps one enter it with a better ear.

Method Atlas

Working supports for the main text. Open an appendix when the chapter points to it. The Atlas is not a standalone textbook, reference work, or protocol.

Appendix A. The DDSRF Case Card

A one-page case formulation through the two-domain grammar of clinical integrability. The central summary instrument of the Method Atlas.

What it is

The DDSRF Case Card is a working case-formulation instrument that gathers all the other DDSRF instruments onto a single page. It is not a diagnostic card, not a treatment plan, and not a case history. It is a card of the current moment: how the client's subjective reality is assembled right now, what holds it, what blocks the next step, and what minimal new experience can be integrated.

The Case Card is re-drawn at every significant point of the work — usually once every few sessions, or at a noticeable shift. It is not made every session: it is a card of a period, not of a momentary state.

When to use

Context	Application
Before starting with a new client	After the first 2–4 sessions, once there is material.
At a standstill in the work	When sessions repeat and there is no movement.
At an unexpected turn	When something has changed substantially.
In supervision	As a basis for reading the case together.
At a handover of responsibility	When the case is passed to another specialist.
Before a significant intervention	When high-load work is planned.

Structure: 12 fields

The Case Card consists of 12 main fields plus one additional. Filling it in takes 15–30 minutes after several sessions with the client.

Field 1. Complaint / situation. What the client brings — in their own words, not in clinical categories. Not "a moderate depressive episode," but "I haven't been able to make myself do anything for three months, everything feels meaningless, I'm not sleeping." This is the entry into the work, not a diagnosis. The client's formulation matters more than the therapist's at this stage.

Field 2. Active phenomenological cluster. The 3–5 invariants now active in the client's experience (Appendix H). Not symptoms and not diagnostic signs, but forms of experience visible in the material: compression of the future, the absence of a lived "I can," flatness of the world, the threat of being seen, the absence of the other, intrusion of the past. A cluster is not one invariant but an interconnected group. Usually 3–5 invariants hold together.

Field 3. Cα mode. Which mode the assembly of the client's subjective reality is now working in (by most sessions, not by the moment): fragmenting, defensively closed, stabilizing, exploratory, transitional (Appendix B). One of the five. If the mode changes across sessions — note the prevailing one and mark the oscillations.

Field 4. Reality weight of the key experience. RW0–RW4 for the main experience that organizes the client's life (Appendix D). Not for all experiences — choose one, the most organizing. State what exactly carries this weight: " 'no one needs me' — RW3" or " 'if I am seen, I will be destroyed' — RW3/RW4." Without specifying which experience carries the weight, the field is useless.

Field 5. Active layers. Which layers of the assembly are now taking part in the current R(t). Of the seven: Pσ, S(t), N(t), B(t), Θ, D_cal, Λ. Usually 3–5 are active. There is no need to mark "all seven active" — it is uninformative.

Field 6. Load-bearing layers. Which of the active layers substantially support the configuration. Without working with them the configuration will not shift. Usually there are 2–3 load-bearing layers. This is not the same as the active ones.

Field 7. Dominant constraint. The main field of the card. Which layer now holds veto power over the next step of change (Appendix C). One layer. Sometimes two. The formulation must be concrete.

> Weak: "trauma"; "attachment"; "cognitive distortions." Strong: "B(t): autonomic hypoactivation against a background of four months without proper sleep; until basic regulation is restored, deep work with traumatic material will be premature."

To the field is attached the strength of the hypothesis: weak (counterfactual test only), medium (counterfactual + one indicator), strong (triangulation — two or three tests converge).

Field 8. What will be premature. Which interventions now look right but will not land. This is a concrete list, not a general principle. For example: "direct work with shame in the room at the current S(t)"; "behavioral experiments at the current level of bodily exhaustion"; "cognitive reframing of the central belief at RW3–RW4." This field guards against premature rightness and against the pressure of the therapist's own school.

Field 9. What must become possible earlier. Which prior condition must be created so that the next step becomes integrable. This is not the next step but the condition for it. For example: "restoration of sleep and basic regulation — three weeks minimum"; "the field as livably-safe — several sessions of tuning pace and presence"; "a distinction of 'then / now' in one concrete situation."

Field 10. Minimal counter-experience. Which small different experience could become the first counter-attractor. Not a "corrective experience" in the broad sense, but a concrete, minimal one, meeting criteria M1–M8 (Appendix F).

> Weak: "help the client feel loved"; "create a corrective experience of safety." Strong: "the client utters a vulnerable statement ('I'm afraid') and lives through the therapist not withdrawing; the first channel of integration is S(t) and the body; then repetition across several sessions."

Field 11. Channels of integration. Through which of the four channels the experience can land (Appendix G): body (a bodily or regulatory trace), relationship (the experience lived with another), narrative (the experience given language), action (the experience linked to a concrete possibility of action). State which channels will be engaged first, which later. Most counter-experiences begin with one or two channels and gradually widen.

Field 12. Counter-load and the field S(t). What this work demands of the therapist. Where the therapist may rush, rescue, retreat, intellectualize, avoid, reinterpret, hurry. This is not self-criticism but a diagnosis of one's own zone of risk. If the therapist does not see the counter-load, he does not work with it, and the field S(t) breaks on the therapist's side. Also — the state of the field S(t): what in the alliance already works; what is fragile; where there were ruptures and how they were repaired.

Field 13 (additional). Epistemic status of the formulation. What in this Case Card is observation, what a working hypothesis, what an open question. This field guards against excessive confidence in the formulation (Appendix K). Use markers: (obs) — observable; (hyp) — hypothesis, requires testing; (open) — open question.

Example of a filled-in Case Card

Client: a man, 38, presenting with a complaint of emotional flattening and doubts about his relationship.

- **1. Complaint:** "I haven't felt anything for my wife for several months. I don't know if I love her. I'm thinking about divorce."
- **2. Active cluster:** emotional flatness; absence of a lived connection; doubt of one's own experience; compression of the future of the relationship.
- **3. Cα mode:** stabilizing, with episodes of defensively closed.
- **4. RW of the key experience:** "I don't feel — so I don't love" — RW3 (obs).
- **5. Active layers:** B(t), N(t), Pσ, S(t).
- **6. Load-bearing layers:** B(t), N(t).
- **7. Dominant constraint:** B(t) (hyp, medium): the client has been taking an antidepressant (SSRI) for six months; the emotional flattening began around the same time; until the medication is adjusted, work on the experience of the relationship will run on distorted material.

- **8. What is premature:** deep work with existential material on the meaning of the relationship; clarifying feelings toward the wife; a decision about divorce.
- **9. What must become possible earlier:** a consultation with a psychiatrist about possible medication adjustment; observation of the change in emotional tone over 2–3 months.
- **10. Minimal counter-experience:** the client acknowledges to himself that the current emotional flatness may be pharmacologically caused and is not equal to a "true" absence of love — without any obligation to decide anything about the marriage now.
- **11. Channels of integration:** first the narrative (a new frame for the state); then action (the consultation); body and relationship later.
- **12. Counter-load:** risk of interpreting this as "a defense against closeness"; risk of working with existential material because it is clinically richer; risk of not referring to a psychiatrist so as "not to disturb the therapeutic relationship"; the field S(t) is still fragile, the client is testing whether I can be trusted.

Use in supervision

The Case Card is an ideal basis for a supervision session. The supervisor asks questions by field:

- Which indicators pointed to this dominant constraint?
- Do two or three tests converge, or is it a weak hypothesis?
- What would an advocate of another school name as dominant?
- What Cα mode was the last session in — and what happened to novelty after your interventions?
- What is the RW of the key experience — and what intervention are you making against that weight?
- What does this work demand of you — where might you hurry, rescue, retreat?

This turns supervision from a discussion of "what I did" into a reading of the moment: what is assembled, what blocks, what is premature, what is possible.

Typical filling errors

Error	What happens
Too many active layers	"All seven active" — the field loses meaning; the distinction between active and load-bearing is erased.
A blurred dominant constraint	"Trauma," "attachment," "cognitive distortions" — without a concrete layer and a concrete blocking mechanism.
A weak hypothesis left unmarked	The therapist works on a weak hypothesis as on a strong one; no triangulation.
Missing "what is premature" field	The therapist records what is possible but not what is not — losing the guard against his own school.
Minimal counter-experience without specifics	Without criteria M1–M8 the field is declarative.
Ignoring the counter-load	The therapist does not see his own zone of risk — the field S(t) is vulnerable.
Epistemic status not stated	A hypothesis is read as a fact; the work runs on false confidence.
The Case Card is not updated	The case moves, the Card stays the same — the formulation goes stale.

The main rule

The Case Card is a working hypothesis about the moment, not a description of the client. The Card does not answer the question "who is this client." The Card answers the question: how is his subjective reality assembled right now, what holds it, what blocks the next step, and what minimal new experience can be integrated.

The Card goes stale. This is normal. The Card is revised. This is part of the work. A therapist whose Case Card does not change for months is either dealing with a stable picture (rare) or has stopped reading it (often).

Final format for printing

For practical use the Case Card can be printed on a single A4 page. Page structure: at the top — the client's name (or code), date filled in, version number; fields 1–13 as brief entries of 2–4 lines each; at the bottom — the date of the next revision. The Card must physically fit on one page. If it does not fit — the formulations are too blurred and need cutting to the essence.

End of Appendix A.

Appendix B. The Cα Mode Map

A working support for Chapter 5. What the system does with novelty at a given moment of the session.

What it is

Cα is the operator that assembles subjective reality. It binds the inputs from all layers — the body, the field of the other, predictive activity, the narrative, history, the coherence thresholds, the context — into a single lived experience. At any moment Cα works in one of five modes. The mode is determined not by what the client says but by what happens to novelty after its contact with the system.

The Mode Map is a working instrument of clinical reading. The therapist asks himself: which mode is the client's assembly of reality working in now? — and on the answer depends what is fit at this minute and what is premature. A detailed discussion of the modes, and of why they describe the moment and not a property of the person, is in Chapter 5.

Three axes through which the mode is read

A mode is a configuration of three parameters of the assembly. Each mode has its own profile.

Axis	Question
Coherence	Is R(t) held as a whole?
Permeability	Can the system take in something new?
Integrability	Can the new become part of experience, not only information?

Five modes: profile across the three axes

Mode	Coherence	Permeability	Integrability
Fragmenting	falling	chaotic	absent
Defensively closed	medium/high	low	almost absent
Stabilizing	growing	cautious	still weak
Exploratory	sufficient	moderate	partial
Transitional	sufficient	high	high but fragile

Mode 1. Fragmenting. *What happens.* Novelty or the current material exceeds the system's coherence. Experience falls apart. *Signs.* Falling coherence of speech — breaks, loss of the thread, a switch to abstraction; panic, emptiness, derealization, disorientation; loss of contact with body, time, place, therapist; inability to hold what was just said; affect exceeds regulatory capacity. *What the therapist does.* Restores coherence through the body, the breath, orientation in the room, the therapist's voice; slows the pace, lowers the intensity; does not interpret, deepen, or explain; holds the field through calm presence. *What he does not do.* Does not ask about emotions or the past; does not offer to "stay with the experience"; does not work with traumatic material; does not use confrontation or exposure.

Mode 2. Defensively closed. *What happens.* Coherence is preserved, but novelty is not let through. Any alternative turns into a confirmation of the old reality or provokes a closing-down. *Signs.* The client speaks coherently but does not become more alive; an intervention turns into proof of the old — "that's exactly what I'm saying"; support is read as a failure to understand; an alternative is quickly devalued; after a good intervention there is more defense, not more space. *What the therapist does.* Does not argue with the content; does not offer an alternative directly; looks for what is being defended by this closure; lowers the threat of novelty — offers less, is present more; works through S(t) — through attunement, pace, the pause. *What he does not do.* Does not insist on the rightness of the intervention; does not repeat the interpretation in other words; does not use "but" against the defense; does not try to "break through" — this strengthens the closure.

Mode 3. Stabilizing. *What happens.* The system is still fragile but takes in support. Novelty does not yet integrate, but coherence grows. *Signs.* The pace slows without closing-down; the client may say "not yet" but not "it's useless"; after regulation there is a little more contact; an intervention does not change deeply but increases what can be held; material can be named without disintegration. *What the therapist does.* Strengthens the body B(t), the field S(t), the coherence thresholds Θ; works at the client's pace; names the state without interpretation; gives space, does not fill the pauses; the main work is to increase capacity, not to bring in new load before its time. *What he does not do.* Does not move to transformational work; does not open material that requires higher coherence thresholds; does not hurry a "breakthrough"; does not confuse stabilization with therapy itself — it is its condition, not its goal.

Mode 4. Exploratory. *What happens.* Curiosity appears. Ambivalence is withstood. Alternative formulations are possible. *Signs.* The client says "maybe," "otherwise," "not sure"; a readiness appears to consider other versions; irony, humor without sarcasm; an ability to hold uncertainty; thoughts begin to widen rather than narrow. *What the therapist does.* Works with distinction — what is the same, what is different; offers alternative formulations; uses thought experiments; makes small behavioral or narrative trials; prepares the ground for a possible counter-experience. *What he does not do.* Does not force a transition to a new experience — that is a different mode; does not confuse intellectual agreement with integration; does not leave the client in this mode too long without movement — there is a risk of "therapy as a beautiful conversation."

Mode 5. Transitional. *What happens.* The old and new reality coexist. A new possibility stops being a thought and begins to be experienced. An ICAE is possible (Appendix G). *Signs.* Affect is strong, but coherence holds; a bodily trace of the new experience appears — the breathing changes, the posture lets go, it becomes possible to stay in contact; the client says "strange," "this is different," "I don't know how to put it"; the old reality is still present but does not seize completely; the moment has a quality of aliveness. *What the therapist does.* Holds the moment without hurrying; helps it integrate through the four channels — body, relationship, narrative, action (Appendix G); names what is happening, but sparely; does not interpret — the experience makes itself; checks that the ICAE does not stay only in the room. *What he does not do.* Does not explain what happened; does not close the moment with a quick generalization; does not turn it into an insight through "so now you see that..."; does not ignore that this mode is fragile — it can roll back within minutes.

Criteria for transitions between modes

Transition	Differential criterion
Fragmenting → Stabilizing	Coherence is restored. The client is reoriented in body, time, contact.
Stabilizing → Exploratory	A “maybe” appears. The client can consider an alternative without closing-down or disintegration.
Exploratory → Transitional	The alternative stops being a thought and begins to be experienced. A bodily trace of the new appears.
Transitional → Fragmenting	Affect has exceeded coherence. Self, other, time, or body lose wholeness.
Exploratory → Defensively closed	An alternative was considered and quickly turned into a threat or devalued.
Defensively closed → Stabilizing	The client stops proving the old reality. There appears: “I can’t go there now, but I’m here.”

The main distinction: defensively closed versus stabilizing

These are the two modes easiest to confuse. Outwardly both can look calm. The difference is fundamental and is read by several signs.

Sign	Defensively closed	Stabilizing
What it does with novelty	rejects	does not yet let through, but does not reject
Reaction to support	support is read as a failure to understand	support is taken in, raises coherence
Dynamics of coherence	coherence is preserved through non-admission	coherence grows through taking in conditions
After the session	repetition of the old position, no widening	a little more can be held
Main marker	after a good intervention — more defense	after a good intervention — more space

> Formula of the distinction: defensive closure preserves the old reality; stabilization increases the possibility of future novelty. This distinction is taken apart in §5.5; here is its working form.

Typical therapist errors by mode

Mode	Typical error
Fragmenting	To continue working with the material that caused the fragmentation.
Defensively closed	To take the defense for a "difficult client" and increase the pressure.
Stabilizing	To confuse stabilization with therapy itself and stay in it endlessly (perpetual stabilization).
Exploratory	To take intellectual agreement for integration.
Transitional	To explain the moment instead of letting it unfold.

Practical rule

The Cα mode is read not by what the client says but by what happens to novelty after its contact with the system. If the therapist can answer the question "what did my last intervention do to the client's system?" — he knows the mode. If he cannot — the mode has not yet been read, and the next intervention will lean more on the habit of one's method than on a reading of the moment.

End of Appendix B.

Appendix C. The Dominant Constraint Protocol

A working support for Chapter 7. What, right now, holds veto power over the next step of change.

What it is

The dominant constraint is the layer of the assembly that at a given moment blocks the next step of change, even if other layers look ready. It is not the deepest source of the problem, not the most noticeable layer of suffering, not the "main trauma" — but what, right now, in this work, makes the next step un-integrable.

The Dominant Constraint Protocol is the main methodological instrument of DDSRF. If the therapist can find the veto, he can read the moment. If he cannot, the work goes by guesswork, even with right interventions. A detailed discussion of the layers and tests is in Chapter 7.

The main question

> What, right now, has the power to stop change, even if everything else looks ready?

Not "what is the root of the problem." Not "what is the main thing." Not "what one usually works with in such clients." But — what blocks the next concrete step. The answer to this question almost always turns out to be one layer, sometimes two.

Three statuses of a layer

Before looking for the veto, one must distinguish three statuses a layer can be in.

Status	What it means
Active layer	Takes part in the current assembly of R(t). Visible in the session.
Load-bearing layer	Substantially supports the configuration. Without it, it does not hold.
Layer with veto power	Blocks the next step of change. Until we work with it, other steps do not land.

This is a critical distinction. Therapists often confuse "what is active" with "where to begin." The active layer is what is visible. The load-bearing one is what holds. The veto is what blocks. These are three different questions.

The seven layers and indicators of veto

Layer	Signs of veto here	What is premature	What must come earlier
B(t) — body	Disturbed sleep, exhaustion, pain; the client "understands" but the body does not follow; after bodily regulation, sharply more availability.	Interpretation, exposure, work with meaning, a demand for action.	Sleep, regulation, medical assessment, bodily steadiness.
S(t) — other/field	A neutral question is experienced as appraisal, a pause as rejection; an intervention breaks not on content but on relationship.	Disclosure of shame, deep interpretation, work with attachment.	Tuning of the field, safety of being seen, repair of contact.
N(t) — narrative	Any new experience is absorbed by the old story: "it's always been this way with me," "this changes nothing."	Behavioral experiments without symbolic processing.	Weakening of the old narrative, a new language, a new frame.
Pσ — predictive activity	Contradicting facts do not update experience; ambiguous signals are steadily read as threat, shame, or rejection.	Rational dissuasion, arguing with the belief.	Lowering the precision of the old prediction through body, field, repeated experience.

Layer	Signs of veto here	What is premature	What must come earlier
Θ — coherence thresholds	On approaching the material, coherence falls: emptiness, derealization, panic, breaks in speech, flight into abstraction.	Transformational work, traumatic material, strong confrontation.	Restoration of coherence, small doses of material, titration.
D_cal — developmental calibration	The present is experienced as the old situation; the reaction is clearly larger than the event; "then" automatically organizes "now."	Work only with the current event.	Recognition of the old calibration, distinction of "then / now," new experience.
Λ — life-world	The real environment keeps producing threat, exhaustion, humiliation, poverty, violence, legal uncertainty.	Inner work without a change of conditions.	Change of conditions, protection, resources, legal or social help.

Three tests for determining the veto

One indicator is a hypothesis. For a hypothesis to become a working one, triangulation is needed: at least two independent sources must point to one layer.

Test 1. The failure test. *Question.* Which right interventions already do not land or strengthen the defense? If the client understands, agrees, but nothing changes — the veto may be at B(t), Pσ, or D_cal. If the client closes precisely in contact — likely at S(t). If any new thought becomes part of the old story — at N(t). If on approaching the theme coherence falls — at Θ. If therapy works in the session but life beyond the door zeroes it all out — at Λ. This is the strongest test, because it is based on an already-observed failure of interventions, not on a hypothesis.

Test 2. The small-support test. *Question.* Which small shift immediately raises coherence or opens access to the work? If grounding, sleep, breath, medical correction, or rest sharply raises the capacity for work — the veto is at the body. If the phrase "we can go slower" returns the client to contact — the veto is at S(t) or Θ. If a new formulation of the story gives space — the veto is at N(t). If a change in the real conditions of life gives more effect than interpretation — the veto is at Λ. This test is almost as strong as Test 1. It rests on an observed effect, not on imagination.

Test 3. The counterfactual test. *Question.* If this layer were temporarily stabilized, would the next step become possible? If yes — it is a candidate for the dominant constraint. If no — the layer is important but does not hold veto power. Example: a client in shame. It seems one must work with the shame. But if one imagines the shame slightly lowered — work is still impossible, because the client sleeps three hours and the body is destroyed. Then right now the veto is at B(t), not at the shame. Important: Test 3 is epistemically weaker than Tests 1 and 2. It is easily infected by the therapist's preferences — a body-oriented therapist will imagine the body is needed; a psychoanalyst, that transference is needed; a CBT therapist, that cognitive work is needed. So it is used third, after Tests 1 and 2.

The rule of triangulation

A veto hypothesis counts as strong only if at least two independent tests point to one layer.

Strength of hypothesis	Basis
Weak	Test 3 only (counterfactual).
Medium	Test 3 + one clinical indicator.
Strong	At least two of the three tests converge on one layer.

Work on a strong hypothesis. A weak one — revise, add information, wait.

The advocate of another school

An additional check for supervision or peer review. Question: which layer would a specialist of another orientation name as dominant?

- A body-oriented therapist — probably the body.
- A psychoanalyst — probably transference (S(t) or D_cal).
- A CBT therapist — probably a schema (N(t) or Pσ).
- A trauma therapist — probably the thresholds or D_cal.
- A systemic therapist — probably S(t) or Λ.

If all the alternative hypotheses converge on one layer, this is strong triangulation. If they diverge, a more attentive reading is needed, and the preferred layer of one's own school becomes the main candidate for revision, not for confirmation. This step guards against theoretical bias: the therapist usually sees what he knows how to work with.

A distinction that is often confused

"Deep source" does not equal "veto now." The dominant constraint is not the root of the problem. It is what blocks the next step. They may coincide, but often do not. A client has a deep developmental trauma (D_cal). That is the root. But right now he is not sleeping, overloaded, in autonomic dysregulation (B(t)). Work with the trauma will be premature. The veto now is at the body. After bodily stabilization the veto may shift. Then D_cal will become the next dominant constraint. But not earlier.

"What is most visible" does not equal "veto now." The most vivid thing in the client's material is often not what blocks movement. A client speaks a great deal about shame. The shame is active. But any work with the shame breaks on S(t): in the therapist's presence the shame only strengthens, because the therapist is experienced as appraising. The active layer is shame (N(t)). The layer with veto power is S(t). First the field needs work, then the shame becomes available.

The rhythm of work with the dominant constraint

The veto is not static. It shifts as the work proceeds.

- Determine the current veto through triangulation.
- Work with it, without ignoring the other layers.
- When the veto lowers, check anew: which layer now blocks the next step?
- The new dominant constraint may turn out to be an entirely different layer.

This does not mean "work with all layers in turn." It means: the veto is a working hypothesis about the next step, not a diagnosis of a layer.

Typical errors

Error	What happens
Confusing the active layer with the veto layer	The therapist works with the most visible material. No effect, because a different layer blocks.
Seeing the veto where you know how to work	The therapist finds the veto in his preferred layer (the body for a body therapist, transference for a psychoanalyst). The defense — triangulation and the advocate of another school.
Working on a weak hypothesis	Only the counterfactual test pointed to a layer. No triangulation. The work goes by guesswork.
Considering the veto permanent	The therapist found the veto and works with it for months, not checking whether it has shifted.
Ignoring Λ	The therapist finds the veto in the inner layers, not noticing that the client lives in a dangerous or destroying environment.
Treating the "root"	The therapist works with the deep trauma as the veto, ignoring that the veto now is on stabilization. The result — fragmentation or closing-down.

Use in case formulation

In the DDSRF Case Card (Appendix A) the dominant constraint is a separate item. The formulation must be concrete.

Weak formulations: "trauma," "shame," "attachment." Strong formulations:

- B(t): autonomic hypoactivation against a background of four months without proper sleep; until basic regulation is restored, deep work with traumatic material will be premature.
- S(t): any intervention requiring the client's visibility is experienced as appraisal; until the field is stabilized as safe, work with shame will strengthen the defense.
- Λ: the client lives with a partner who continues psychological violence; inner work on self-worth is zeroed out by the external context and may strengthen the sense of personal inadequacy.

Practical rule

The dominant constraint has been found when working with it increases the possibility of the next step, and bypassing it makes the next step premature. This is not a philosophical assumption but a clinical check of the moment. If the hypothesis is right, space appears in the work. If it is wrong, no space appears, and a different hypothesis is needed.

End of Appendix C.

Appendix D. The RW0–RW4 Scale and Clinical Grid of Application

A working support for Chapter 6. Not a diagnostic instrument and not a point-score — an instrument for the clinical reading of the reality weight of a particular experience.

D.1. How to use the RW scale

Reality weight (RW) describes how far a particular experience acts as reality for the client — how far it organizes the body, attention, action, and how resistant it is to refutation. The five-level scale (RW0–RW4) is a working distinction, not a measurement. Before using it, one must hold five defenses, without which it immediately turns into a hidden typology or a protocol of technique.

- RW belongs to the experience, not the client. One cannot write "the client is RW3." One can write "the experience 'I am unloved' now has RW3" or "the experience 'if I ask, I will be humiliated' holds RW4." In the same client at one moment, different experiences carry different weight.
- RW is not measured in points. The level is read by a combination of signs — bodily trace, effect on action, resistance to refutation — not computed. It is a qualitative map, not a scale.
- RW does not equal truth. High weight does not mean the experience is objectively correct. It means it acts as reality.
- RW does not equal the intensity of affect. A quiet, level hopelessness can have high RW; a stormy emotion, low. The loud is not always weighty.
- RW is not a protocol for choosing a technique. It shows which forms of work usually become more available or more dangerous. The final

fit is still decided through capacity, load, the Cα mode, the dominant constraint, and the field — not by the RW level itself.

The scale answers not the question "is the client right" but the question "what is now possible to do with this experience at all." It is an instrument of clinical reading, not of judgment about content.

D.2. RW0–RW4: a qualitative scale

Five recognizable degrees of how far an experience acts as reality. Each level is given as a card: definition, how to hear, what is usually available, frequent error.

RW0. Semantic content. *Definition.* The content is there as words: the client utters a phrase, describes, agrees with an idea — but it stays words. No bodily trace, no change in action, no presence beyond the conversation. *How to hear.* In speech — an even sayability without echo, an easy switch to the opposite without resistance. In the body — no trace. In the field — the content does not "settle." In action — no change. Example: "Yes, I suppose I deserve love, like everyone" — level, without a pause, without a trace in the next few minutes. *What is usually available.* Discussion, informing, psychoeducation, clear definitions, clarification of concepts — all that stays at the level of content. *Frequent error.* To take uttered content for integration. Agreement at RW0 does not equal a change of weight; a week later the client returns to where he was.

RW1. Possible perspective. *Definition.* The idea is admitted as one of the possible ones: the client considers, compares, weighs. There is intellectual interest, but no stable bodily trace yet; the idea is held in the conversation but does not govern, and without a reminder does not return between sessions. *How to hear.* In speech — "maybe," "I allow for it," an even tone without a shift. In the body — a fleeting echo, not taking hold. In the field — an exploratory intonation. In action — no stable changes. Example: "I thought about what you said. Maybe I really am too hard on myself. Not sure, but I allow for it." *What is usually available.* Cognitive work, reframing, discussion in the exploratory Cα mode, small behavioral trials, hypotheses. *Frequent error.* To take "maybe" for "already become." An idea at RW1 is not yet reality; it is premature to build work on it as on an achieved shift.

RW2. Situational reality. *Definition.* The experience becomes real in particular contexts: in some situations it governs, in others not. It is trigger-dependent. Outside the trigger the client often speaks of it at a distance and can predict where it will "hit." *How to hear.* In speech — a calm description outside the trigger and a sharp change of tone in trigger situations. In the body — a trace appears in particular contexts. In the field — the presence of the experience now arises, now leaves. Example: in the room the client calmly tells of a criticizing boss — but in a meeting in his presence experiences himself as worthless, cannot speak, the body contracts. *What is usually available.* Work with concrete triggers, bodily work at the moment of onset, relational work in the room as a reproduction, safe micro-trials in concrete contexts. *Frequent error.* To generalize to the whole of life what now weighs situationally — and to work "too globally," losing the point of application. Or the reverse, to miss the transition from situational to dominant weight.

RW3. Dominant reality. *Definition.* The experience governs the body, attention, and action despite rational disagreement. The client notices the gap himself — "I understand, but I experience it otherwise." The bodily trace is stable or frequently recurring; the experience is present in most contexts and directs the choice of relationships, work, behavior. Rational refutation does not land. *How to hear.* In speech — "I understand, but...," "I know it's not so, yet I live as if it were." In the body — a stable presence. In the field — the experience organizes contact. In action — it determines choices. Earlier interventions bring back the same reaction. *What is usually available.* Reading the dominant constraint (Appendix C), a sequence of steps, a minimal counter-experience with a load carefully matched to capacity, work with the layers of the assembly. *Frequent error.* To treat RW3 as RW1 — to argue, persuade, present facts, count agreement as a drop in weight. At this level cognitive restructuring without work on the layers does not land; an exchange of facts strengthens the defense or goes into pseudo-agreement.

RW4. Self-sealed reality. *Definition.* The experience becomes almost impermeable to refutation. All incoming data are interpreted in its favor, alternatives do not land, the system self-confirms. Contradicting facts are reinterpreted to fit the old reality; confirmations are found even where there are none; rational criticism is perceived as a threat. Such a reality has a quality of compulsion. *How to hear.* In speech — all facts fit into one and the same reading, any neutral phrase receives the same sign. In the body — a stable organizing presence. In the field — support is read as threat or pity, neutrality as confirmation of the worst. Example: the client is certain his colleagues despise him — and any neutral phrase becomes hidden contempt, any support is read as pity, any absence of reaction as confirmation that he does not deserve attention. *What is usually available.* First — stabilization, safety, risk assessment, work with the body and basic conditions. If necessary — a psychiatric referral and specialized assessment. Direct work with content at this level is not merely useless — it is perceived as an attack. *Frequent error.* Not to distinguish severe neurotic self-sealing from a possible shift toward O4–O5 (see D.4). And the second, symmetrical one: to treat RW4 as RW3 through insight and argument, without first changing the task to stabilization.

D.3. The clinical grid: what is usually available at each level

A summary grid matching RW levels to available work. This is not a prescription of technique-choice but a guide: what most often lands at this level, what is often premature, and the main error the reading slips into. The final fit is always decided on the concrete material.

RW	What the level shows	What is usually available	What is often premature	Main error
RW0	Content is there as words, no trace in body and action	Discussion, informing, psychoeducation, clear definitions	To expect a change of body, relationship, action from the uttered	To take uttered content for integration
RW1	The idea is admitted as a possibility	Exploration, cognitive work, small behavioral trials, hypotheses	To consider the idea already become reality	To take “maybe” for “already become”
RW2	The experience is real in particular contexts	Trigger-specific work, the body in the moment, safe micro-trials	To generalize to the whole of life, to work “too globally”	To work without a point of application; to miss the transition to RW3
RW3	The experience acts as a dominant reality	Dominant constraint, sequence, minimal counter-experience	Argument, facts, direct persuasion, insight-work without layers	To treat the experience as a thought, to count agreement as a drop in weight

RW	What the level shows	What is usually available	What is often premature	Main error
RW4	The experience self-confirms, alternatives do not land	First safety, stabilization, risk assessment; specialized assessment as indicated	Work with content as with a discussable idea	Not to distinguish severe self-sealing from a shift toward O4–O5

The grid is read by rows, but the decision is never made by it alone. In parallel one reads the Cα mode (Appendix B), the dominant constraint (Appendix C), load, capacity, and field (Appendix E). The same RW level requires different work under different modes and different vetoes — the grid shows a zone, it does not prescribe a move.

D.4. Frequent errors in reading RW

- To ascribe RW to the client, not to the experience. "He is RW4" is a category error: it is the experience in the moment that has weight, not the person. In the same client "I am loved" may weigh little, "I am unloved" much.
- To confuse RW with the intensity of affect. The loud is not always weighty. A quiet hopelessness can have high RW; a stormy emotion, low. Read the combination of signs, not the loudness.
- To confuse RW with truth. What weighs as reality is not necessarily objectively true — and vice versa. Reading the weight answers "what is possible to do with this," not "is the client right."
- To take agreement for a drop in RW. The client understood, nodded, said it through — this does not mean the experience changed. It means the content shifted to RW0–RW1; the old high-weight reality may have stayed untouched.
- To work with RW3/RW4 through arguments. Argument raises the defense or goes into pseudo-agreement. At high levels what is needed is work with the layers and a minimal counter-experience, not an exchange of facts.
- Not to see the boundary of safety at RW4. Self-sealing touches reality testing — that is already the zone O4–O5: dissociative fragmentation or psychotic disorganization. Specialized clinical assessment

comes first, not work with the weight. RW4 ≠ psychosis, but with a disturbance of reality testing it is a different clinical situation.

- To use RW as a protocol of technique. RW helps read fit but does not replace the Cα mode, the dominant constraint, load/capacity, and field. The grid D.3 is a guide, not a prescription.

D.5. How to record RW in the Case Card

In the DDSRF Case Card (Appendix A) reality weight is recorded not as a score for the client but as a characteristic of a particular experience, with reference to the signs and the consequences for the work. The recording format is short — experience, level, signs, consequence.

Example 1. Experience: "if I am seen, I will be destroyed." RW: RW3. Signs: the body contracts under a gaze, a stable avoidance of being seen; the client rationally understands that no destruction occurs but acts out of threat; the experience returns in most contact situations. Consequence: directly naming the shame and praise are premature. What is needed is a minimal experience of safe visibility — the experience that here one can be seen and not judged (link to CCP-4, P-IN2).

Example 2. Experience: "this random detail is addressed to me." RW: RW4; check for a shift toward O4–O5. Signs: alternatives do not land, coincidences self-confirm, the reality-check shared with another is disturbed; rational doubt quickly fades. Consequence: first comes an assessment of the stability of the assembly and of safety (boundary P-IN1, P-SA3). Work with content at this level is premature.

Example 3. Experience: "I may not come close." RW: appeared at RW1, held over two sessions. Signs: the idea is admitted as a possibility, the bodily trace so far episodic; in one situation it was experienced from the body as a real option. Consequence: the counter-experience is fragile — it is premature to load it with an obligation or to fix it as "achieved." Help the restored agency (P-AG3) pass through the four channels — body, contact, word, small action — so that it gains a path to repetition.

The Case Card entry is made in the language of the client's experience, not in the abstract language of the configuration. This holds the discipline of D.1: RW belongs to a particular experience, not to the person.

End of Appendix D.

Appendix E. The Load–Capacity–Field Grid

The fit of integration load, integrative capacity, and the field of meeting. A working support for Chapter 4.

What it is

This is the central instrument for applying the principle of clinical integrability. It answers the question: is this intervention fit now? The answer depends not on the quality of the intervention and not on its content. It depends on whether its load fits the current capacity of the system — the client, the therapist, and the field between them.

Three quantities and the counter-load

Quantity	What it describes
Integration load	What this intervention demands of the client — what material he must withstand, hold, process, include in his reality.
Integrative capacity	What the client can now take in without defensive closure, fragmentation, or pseudo-agreement.
Field S(t)	What is now possible between client and therapist — how far the field withstands this work.
Counter-load	What this intervention demands of the therapist — what affect, shame, uncertainty, urge to rescue or interpret he must withstand.

The main principle

An intervention is fit when the load fits the capacity — of the client, the therapist, and the field. Not "right in content." Not "theoretically grounded." Not "consistent with the school." But — fits the capacity.

This is the basis of clinical integrability. Everything else in DDSRF is instruments for assessing this fit. A detailed discussion is in §4.4–4.5.

Three zones of the ratio

Zone	Ratio	What happens
Underload	load < capacity	Work is safe but does not change the configuration. Therapy becomes supportive or stagnant.
Fit	load ≈ capacity	An optimal tension appears. A counter-attractor and ICAE become possible.
Overload	load > capacity	Defensive closure, fragmentation, retraumatization, pseudo-agreement, or dropout.

All three states can be a clinical error. Overload is the obvious one. Underload is less obvious but no less real. A therapist who endlessly stabilizes "so as not to harm" gradually creates perpetual stabilization — a state in which the client stays safe but does not change.

What determines the integration load of an intervention

Factor	Description
Depth	How close to the core of the configuration the intervention works.
Strength of the counter-attractor	How strongly the intervention contradicts the reality weight of the old configuration.
Opening of material	Whether the work requires opening closed material (trauma, shame, early losses).
Visibility	Whether the work requires being seen by the therapist.
Action	Whether the work requires going beyond habitual action.
Affective density	How much affect may be evoked.

Factor	Description
Duration of contact with the material	How long one must stay with the material for the intervention to work.

What determines the client's integrative capacity

Factor	Description
Cα mode	Fragmenting and defensively closed — low capacity. Exploratory and transitional — high.
Coherence thresholds Θ	How far the client can hold the wholeness of experience under load.
B(t) — body	Sleep, regulation, energy, medical conditions.
S(t) — field	How far the other is experienced as safe or dangerous.
RW of the old configuration	The higher the RW, the stronger the new intervention must be to land.
D_cal — old calibration	How far the present is already seized by old expectations.
Λ — external context	Whether the environment is destroying what is being created in the room.

What determines the counter-load on the therapist

This is the part most often ignored. Yet an intervention works only if the therapist can withstand it.

Factor	Description
Affective density	How far the therapist must withstand the affect without turning away.
The client's shame	Whether the therapist can witness shame without the urge to comfort, fix, turn away.
The pause	Whether the therapist can be silent when he wants to fill it.
Uncertainty	Whether the therapist can not know what will happen next.
Countertransference	Whether the therapist can hold his own reactions (rescue, judgment, hopelessness) without acting from them.
Pace	Whether the therapist can go at the client's pace, without hurrying.
Helplessness	Whether the therapist can be beside what he cannot change.

If the therapist does not withstand the counter-load, the field breaks on the therapist's side, even if the technique is flawless.

What determines the capacity of the field S(t)

The field is the third participant in the intervention. It has its own capacity.

Factor	Description
Established alliance	How far working trust has formed.
History of ruptures and repair	Whether there has been rupture/repair experience, or the field is still untested.
Session pace	Whether there is enough time in this session for this work.
External conditions	Therapist fatigue, noise, interruptions, format (online or offline).
Pace alignment	Whether the paces of client and therapist coincide or are out of sync.

Load benchmarks of typical interventions

These are benchmarks, not a rigid scale. The same type of intervention may have different load in different clients.

Intervention	Load for the client	Counter-load	Required field capacity
Reflection of experience	low	low	basic
Normalization of the state	low	low	basic
Psychoeducation	low	low	basic
Cognitive reframing	medium	medium	stable field
Behavioral experiment	medium	medium	stable field
Work with triggers	medium/high	medium	reliable field
Psychoanalytic interpretation	medium/high	medium/high	worked-through transference
Small exposure	medium/high	medium/high	reliable field
Work with defenses	high	high	reliable field
Work with shame in the presence of another	very high	very high	deep alliance
Traumatic processing	very high	very high	specialized training
Direct confrontation	very high	very high	deep alliance
Work with the collapse of meaning	very high	very high	the therapist's ability to withstand

The main rule of fit

The choice of intervention is not the choice of the "right" technique. It is the choice of an intervention whose load fits the capacity. A technically right intervention under overload does not land. A technically less precise intervention under fit lands and works. This is not a justification of "weak" interventions. It is a methodological rule: rightness is determined not only by content but by integrability.

When to increase load, when to lower it

Increase load when:

- Cα is in the exploratory or transitional mode.
- The coherence thresholds Θ are stable.
- B(t) gives resource.
- S(t) is reliable.
- Previous interventions integrated easily — there is a reserve of capacity.
- The work is stagnating at one level (risk of perpetual stabilization).
- The client himself signals readiness — "we can go further," "I'm ready to look deeper."

Lower load when:

- Cα is in the defensively closed or fragmenting mode.
- The coherence thresholds Θ are falling.
- B(t) is exhausted.
- S(t) is breaking — the therapist is experienced as dangerous.
- The previous intervention caused closing-down or fragmentation.
- Signs of pseudo-agreement appear.
- The therapist feels that he himself cannot withstand it — the counter-load exceeds his capacity.

Signs of overload

In the client:

- Sudden closing-down, withdrawal, formal answers.
- Falling coherence of speech.
- Loss of contact with the body or with the therapist.
- Autonomic activation — tachycardia, tremor, pallor.
- Pseudo-agreement — too quick, too smooth.
- Dissociative signs.
- A wish to break off the session.

In the therapist:

- A wish to rescue, comfort, fix — as a signal that the load is high.
- A wish to distance, explain, interpret.
- An inner acceleration, a wish to "make progress."
- A sense that "it's time to do something."

In the field:

- The rhythm of the session breaks.
- Ruptures appear that do not repair naturally.
- The pace speeds up or sharply slows.

On detecting any of these signs — lower the load. Do not explain, do not interpret. Return to a simpler level of work: body, orientation, contact, simple presence.

Signs of under-load

- The work stagnates, sessions become repetitive.
- The client is comfortable but the configuration does not change.
- A sense appears that sessions are "pleasant but not moving."
- The client speaks of significant themes outside the session and does not bring them inside.
- ICAE does not arise, because the tension for it is insufficient.
- The therapist feels that "something must change, but I'm afraid."

On detecting this — increase the load. Not sharply. But add density: a more precise formulation, a deeper question, a more open break in the narrative.

Two symmetrical errors

Error	What happens
Premature rightness	A technically right intervention at a load above capacity. Result — closing-down, fragmentation, pseudo-agreement.
Perpetual stabilization	Chronic maintenance of capacity without checking its growth. Result — stagnation, absence of change.

Both errors are equally dangerous clinically. DDSRF is a theory of fit, not a theory of caution.

Use in case formulation

In the DDSRF Case Card (Appendix A) there are three linked items:

- Current capacity. At what level the client's ability to integrate the new stands.
- Load of the planned intervention. What this work demands.
- Counter-load. What this work demands of the therapist — where he may hurry, rescue, retreat, intellectualize.

If these three items do not fit one another, the intervention needs correction.

Practical rule

Before every significant intervention the therapist asks himself three questions:

- What will this work demand of the client — can he withstand it now?
- What will this work demand of me — can I withstand it now?
- What will the field between us withstand now?

If the answer to any of the three is "no" or "not sure" — the intervention needs preparation, not execution.

End of Appendix E.

Appendix F. Criteria of the Minimal Counter-Experience

A working support for Chapter 9. Eight criteria distinguishing a minimal counter-experience from insight, catharsis, agreement, and a strong session.

F.1. What a minimal counter-experience is

A minimal counter-experience is the smallest lived experience of a different organization of reality that already differs from the old configuration but does not yet exceed the current integrative capacity of the client, the therapist, and the field. Not an explanation that another reality is possible, but a small patch of that other reality, actually occurred in the moment.

Before using the criteria, one must hold the defenses without which the application turns into a manual on "how to create a counter-experience" — which is exactly what Chapter 9 calls forcing.

- Not a technique. A counter-experience is not created by the force of an intervention and not summoned by a device. It becomes possible when the load of the new falls into the zone of fit with the current capacity.
- Not an exercise and not exposure. A set exposure may become a counter-experience — or break the assembly. The setting-up itself guarantees nothing; fit decides, not the structure of the task.
- Not an insight. Insight changes the map, counter-experience changes the availability of the territory. "I understood" is not a counter-experience; "I said something vulnerable and was not rejected" is.

- Not a strong emotion. The force of affect does not equal a counter-experience: a storm may roar through without shifting anything; a quiet moment may shift it.
- Not the goal of every session. Most of the work is work with conditions: reading the moment, sequence, capacity, field. A counter-experience happens on this ground when it is ready.
- Not a "breakthrough." A minimal counter-experience is by definition small. The search for dramatic events usually passes by the change that goes through the small.

The formula that holds the whole appendix: a minimal counter-experience is not created by the force of an intervention — it becomes possible when the load of the new falls into the zone of fit with the current capacity of the client, the therapist, and the field.

F.2. The eight criteria M1–M8

Eight signs by whose combination a minimal counter-experience is told from its look-alikes. Six main ones are named in Chapter 9; M1 (relative minimality) and M2 (correspondence to the current Cα mode) are set out separately as conditions, without which the other six cannot be read precisely.

M1. Relative minimality. The experience is minimal not by external size but in relation to the system's current capacity. For one client a minimal step is to raise the eyes to the therapist; for another, to speak before a group. "Minimal" is a technical characteristic, meaning "small enough to land, but different enough from the old configuration to be new."

M2. Correspondence to the current Cα mode. A counter-experience is possible within the current mode of assembly or at its nearest border. In the defensively closed mode one cannot force a transitional moment; first the load of novelty must be lowered, the assembly allowed into the stabilizing or exploratory mode. A counter-experience that does not correspond to the mode either does not land or brings down coherence.

M3. Livedness, not explanation. A counter-experience has the quality of "this happened," not "I understood." Not "I understood that I am not rejected," but "I said something vulnerable and was not rejected." If the experience stays at the level of formulation, not engaging the body, the field, and action, it is an insight, not a counter-experience. The distinction continues directly from Chapter 9.2: insight changes the map, counter-experience changes the availability of the territory.

M4. Bodily or regulatory trace. There must be at least a small bodily or regulatory trace. Not necessarily a "vivid body" — but something changed: breathing, a pause, a relaxation of the shoulders, support, a decrease of tightening, access to the body, stabilization, silence instead of the former mobilization. Without some trace in the body a counter-experience stays an event in speech and quickly fades.

M5. Indirect work with the old reality. A counter-experience does not attack the old reality head-on and does not say "you are wrong." It creates a small lived fact that the old configuration cannot absorb at once, without assaulting it frontally. Direct refutation at high reality weight (RW3–RW4) does not work; a counter-experience bypasses the argument and creates an experience that the old logic does not manage to rewrite in its favor.

M6. The old configuration does not become more convincing. After a counter-experience the old configuration may temporarily activate — this is part of normal oscillation (see G.4). But if it has become more sealed, more convincing, gained new confirmation — this is not a counter-experience but a reinforcement of it. The sign of a real counter-experience is that the old does not strengthen; the sign of a look-alike or of prematureness is that the old is assembled more densely after the event.

M7. Potential repeatability. A counter-experience must have a path to repetition, at least in close situations. If it is possible only as a unique dramatic episode, not reproducible in ordinary conditions, it may be a strong session but not the beginning of structural change. Not repetition itself — but a real possibility of repetition in something close.

M8. Minimal nameability. The experience can be named by the client in his own words — not at once and not precisely, but somehow. "Strange, but I didn't fall through"; "I managed a little"; "there's a bit more room." The words need not be accurate, but a counter-experience usually finds them. If the experience left no trace in speech at all, it risks not integrating into the narrative.

The criteria M1–M8 are read by combination, not separately. One or two matching signs is more likely a look-alike (see F.3). A real minimal counter-experience leaves a cumulative trace along several lines at once.

F.3. Look-alikes of the counter-experience

A minimal counter-experience has several convincing look-alikes, and if they are not distinguished, the work can go the wrong way for months. This continues §9.7 directly.

- Insight. A new map. "I've got it!" with elation, but the experience did not enter the body and stayed at the level of formulation. It changes what the client knows, not what he experiences.
- Shift of state. It became easier, warmer, clearer, calmer. Real, but it may vanish by evening. It does not distinguish itself from bodily-affective relief, has no repeatability, and often leaves no trace in action.
- Catharsis. A strong affective discharge — tears, rage, a breakthrough. It feels like a huge event, but a week later all is as it was. The force of affect does not equal a counter-experience; a storm may roar through without shifting anything.
- Pseudo-agreement. The client agreed with the therapist's formulation — perhaps sincerely — but this is agreement with someone else's words, not his own lived experience. "Pseudo-" here means not the client's insincerity but the absence of integration and of a change of weight. It changes what the client says, not what he experiences.
- Strong session. A subjectively powerful event in the room without repeatability in ordinary life. One or two signs of a real counter-experience — but not the cumulative trace.
- Single counter-experience. A real minimal counter-experience took place but has not yet passed through the channels of integration. This is not yet ICAE (see Appendix G); what separates the one from the other is there.

The main formula of the distinction: a look-alike resembles a counter-experience by one or two signs. A real minimal counter-experience leaves a cumulative trace — in the experience, the body, the field, the word, and the possibility of repetition.

F.4. What is often premature

This section is needed so that F is not read as "how to create a counter-experience." Typical prematurenesses that turn a possible counter-experience into a look-alike or into a collapse of the assembly:

- Making the counter-experience too large — exposure or an intervention beyond the current capacity; M1 is violated, and the experience either does not land or breaks coherence.
- Turning the counter-experience into a technique — setting oneself the task of "evoking an ICAE" this session; forcing closes the very thing the therapist is after.
- Fixing it in words before the experience is lived — "so now you see…": the experience turns back into an insight, into a map, losing precisely what made it territory.
- Rejoicing for the client before he himself has withstood the new experience — to celebrate at the moment when the experience is still fragile is to load it with expectation and often to cut it off.
- Demanding repetition — turning a small shift into an obligation "now do this every day"; M7 is about the possibility of repetition, not about forcing it.
- Turning a small experience into a plan — expanding it to goals and obligations; the early form does not hold such weight and returns to collapse.
- Praise, if it increases exposure — for a shame organization (CCP-4, P-IN2) praise is read as one more appraisal and closes what has just opened.
- Going to action before the new experience has gained a body and a field — without M4 and M3, action has no ground and quickly rolls back.

F.5. Three examples of a minimal counter-experience

Brief examples showing how M1–M8 work on concrete configurations. These are not models to reproduce but illustrations of the distinction.

CCP-4 (shame organization of the self). The minimal counter-experience is a small visibility without added shame: a moment in which the client is seen and not appraised, not comforted too quickly, not corrected. M3 — lived, not said: "you looked, and I was not destroyed." M4 — a bodily trace: the shoulders dropped, the breathing changed. M5 — the old shame is not attacked directly. M6 — after the moment the old configuration did not become more convincing. M7 — repetition is possible in a small dose in the following sessions.

CCP-1 (compression of the future). The minimal counter-experience is a small gap between "now" and "later": one experience in which the future unfolds, for a second, by one step. M3 — lived: not a built plan but a sense of extension. M4 — bodily: "it released in the chest." M1 — minimal in relation to capacity: not "a plan for the year" but a small step in the time perspective.

CCP-8 (noetic overload). The minimal counter-experience is an experience of the neutral: a moment in which a detail can stay in the background, not loaded with meaning. M3 — lived as a rest from meaning, not "a new meaning." M5 — not an argument with the salience, but its lowering through the experience of the neutral. M2 — corresponds to the stability of the assembly (at a shift toward O4–O5 safety comes first, not work with the form).

F.6. Transition to Appendix G

A minimal counter-experience is not the end of change. It is an event that can become its beginning. A counter-experience is fragile: it may take place and not take hold, may roll back within minutes, may stay a single episode without a trace in life. For it to become the beginning of a structural shift, it must pass through the four channels — body, field/relationship, narrative, action — and gain repeatability over time.

This is what Appendix G deals with: the micro-dynamics of integration (I0–I5), oscillations between the old configuration and the new experience, the three indicators of consolidation, and the durability-of-change scale (L1–L4). F answers the question "what counts as a minimal counter-experience"; G answers the question "when it becomes integrated and begins to take hold."

End of Appendix F.

Appendix G. The ICAE Map: Integration, Oscillations, and the Durability of Change

A working support for Chapter 9. Two axes (I0–I5 and L1–L4), four channels of integration, oscillations, three indicators of consolidation.

G.1. What ICAE is

ICAE — the Integrated Counter-Attractor Experience: a counter-experience that has begun to enter the four channels of life. It is not a stronger counter-experience, not a dramatic moment, and not a "consolidation technique." It is a counter-experience that did not stay at one point but resonated in the body, the field, the word, and action enough to gain a path to repetition.

> The formula that holds the whole appendix: a counter-experience becomes ICAE not because it was strong but because it was held enough and began to enter several channels of life.

Defenses without which ICAE immediately turns into the goal of a technique:

- ICAE need not be dramatic. Change often goes through small moments that do not look like an event. The search for vivid events misses the integration that goes quietly.
- ICAE is not created by technique. The therapist does not produce ICAE and does not summon it by a device. He creates the conditions, notices the moment when a counter-experience begins to hold, and helps it not to fall apart.

- ICAE is not the goal of every session. Most of the work is work with conditions. ICAE happens on this ground when it is ready; forcing closes what the therapist is after.
- One ICAE ≠ structural change. ICAE is an event on the micro-dynamics axis (I), not an achievement on the durability axis (L). Between "an ICAE happened in the room today" and "the client's life has changed" there are usually weeks or months of work.

G.2. The four channels of integration

A counter-experience begins to take hold when it resonates not at one point but in several channels. There are four, and they are not hierarchical: none is "more important," and not all four necessarily activate at once — but a counter-experience that stayed in only one channel usually stays fragile.

- Body. A regulatory trace appeared: a change of breathing, a pause, support, tone, access to the body, a decrease of tightening. Not a "vivid body," but something changed bodily.
- Field / relationship. The new experience was withstood with another: contact did not break at the moment of vulnerability, the field held the moment without drawing-in and without withdrawal. The counter-experience passed the test by another.
- Narrative / word. The client can name what happened in his own words — even approximately. "I said it, and you didn't turn away"; "strange, but I didn't fall through." The word need not be precise, but a counter-experience usually finds it.
- Action. At least a small path into life appears — not a plan, but a real possibility of repetition in something close. Once did not hide; once said "no"; one micro-movement toward the new.

A running example holding the appendix (CCP-4, P-IN2). The client said something vulnerable for the first time in the session; the therapist stayed in contact. Body: the breathing changed, the shoulders dropped. Field: contact withstood, without drawing-in and without appraisal. Narrative: "I said it, and you didn't turn away." Action: the next week at work he once did not hide behind a manager's general question. Four channels — four places where the new gained a trace.

G.3. I0–I5: the micro-dynamics of integration

The first axis — what happened in the moment and between sessions. Six recognizable steps; read by a combination of signs, not by the client's words.

- I0. Explanation. The client understood a new thought or received a frame. The content is there as words. Not yet change.
- I1. Shift of state. It became easier, clearer, warmer, calmer. Real, but it may vanish by evening. Without a trace in action it does not take hold.
- I2. First counter-experience. The client lived through a small patch of a different reality. The beginning of structural change. A fragile event, not yet passed through the channels of integration.
- I3. ICAE. The new possibility was lived and held through the four channels: body, relationship, narrative, action. The counter-experience gained a cumulative trace; now it has a chance of repetition.
- I4. Repeated availability. The experience is reproduced not only in the room — first with intimates, then in wider contexts. Not every time and not everywhere, but the new reality becomes summonable.
- I5. Recalibration. The old configuration loses the status of the main reality; D_cal updates. The new no longer requires an effort of holding; it has become part of how the assembly works by default.

The scale is read as a direction, not as linear progress: between the steps rollbacks are possible, and I5 is already a zone of durability (see G.6), not of one session. The main thing: I0 and I1 are not a counter-experience; I2 is the first counter-experience, not yet ICAE; I3 is ICAE; I4–I5 are consolidation and the shift of the old attractor.

G.4. Oscillations of integration

The most important thing to know about how change proceeds — it does not go in a straight line. It goes through oscillations between the old configuration and the new counter-experience.

The typical picture. In the session — a real ICAE, held through the body and contact (I3). Between sessions the old reality takes over again: the client remembers the relief but lives again as before (a rollback to I1 or even I0). In the next session a small counter-experience happens again (I2). After several such cycles I4 appears — the ability to summon the new experience beyond the room. The old does not leave at once — it has years of history, and one episode of the new cannot instantly displace it.

This must be said plainly. A rollback after ICAE does not mean the ICAE was false. It is the normal form of the movement of integration. A therapist who, at the first rollback, decides "it didn't work" and changes tactics cuts off the very oscillation that is the mechanism of consolidation. A rollback by itself is not a signal to change course; often it is part of the course.

But the character of the rollbacks must be read. The defense against the opposite error: if rollbacks become deeper, more dangerous, or last longer — this is no longer normal oscillation but a reason to reconsider the load, the field, or the sequence. Normal oscillation decreases in amplitude and lengthens in the intervals between rollbacks. A growing, deepening oscillation is a signal that something in the work is not being withstood.

G.5. Three indicators of ICAE consolidation

What tells us that change is really consolidating? Not the absence of rollbacks — they are to be expected — but a change in their character. Three signs, read over time.

- Speed of return. If before, after a rollback, the client returned to the new experience over weeks, now it is days, then hours. The shortening of recovery time is the main sign of consolidation.
- Breadth of transfer. The new experience appears no longer only in the room — first with intimates, then with strangers, then on its own. Not "everywhere and always," but a widening of the zones where the new is available.
- Waning power of the old. The old reality still rises but no longer seizes the whole; the client notices the old experience without getting lost in it. A lowering of the reality weight of the old configuration (see Appendix D).

These three signs are read together and gradually. One of them without the other two is a weak support. All three, appearing over time, say that the oscillation is really shifting the assembly, not just oscillating in place.

G.6. L1–L4: the durability of change

The second axis answers a different question: how far the change has taken hold over time. This is not "what happened in the moment" (the I axis) but "how far the new has become an available alternative to the old." Four steps, read on a scale of weeks and months.

- L1. Momentary shift of state. Experienced differently once; not reproduced on its own. The experience took place but is held only in the room and only with the support of the field.
- L2. Repeatable availability. The experience can be summoned deliberately; it works under certain conditions. The client knows the new is possible and can sometimes turn to it — but it requires effort and a suitable context.
- L3. Weakening of the old attractor. The old configuration loses force; the alternative is comparable in availability. The new is no longer a rare event; the old is no longer the only reality. This is already a structural shift.
- L4. Durable revision of calibration. The new organization of experience has become part of ordinary life; D_cal is updated. The old configuration may activate at times but no longer sets "how things are by default." This is a zone of stable change, not of an event.

The main error of the therapist on this axis is to take I3 for L3. Between a strong session with ICAE and a weakening of the old attractor there are usually weeks or months of work. ICAE is an event on the micro-dynamics axis, L3 a state on the durability axis; they cannot be collapsed. A therapist who confuses these axes takes a vivid session for recovery and is then puzzled why a week later the client is "as he was." He is not as he was: one counter-experience took place. But one counter-experience is an event on the first axis, not an achievement on the second.

G.7. Frequent errors in work with ICAE

- To take insight for ICAE. "I've got it!" with elation is I0 (explanation), not I3. Without a trace in body, field, action it is a map, not a territory.

- To take a shift of state for ICAE. “It became easier” is I1, not I3. It may vanish by evening without transfer into the channels of integration.
- To take one ICAE for stable change. To confuse I3 with L3 (see G.6). Between them are usually weeks or months.
- To explain the moment instead of letting it unfold. “So now you see…” turns a counter-experience back into an insight.
- To rejoice or celebrate for the client prematurely. It loads a fragile experience with expectation and often cuts it off; for a shame organization it increases exposure.
- To demand repetition. To turn a small shift into an obligation “now do this every day”; repeatability as a condition, not as coercion.
- Not to track action in life. Without the fourth channel ICAE stays an event of the room; life does not change, and the change does not take hold.
- Not to see a rollback as normal oscillation. To change tactics at the first rollback is to cut off the mechanism of consolidation.
- Not to reconsider the load when rollbacks become dangerous. The symmetrical error: to consider any rollback normal when the oscillation is no longer decreasing but growing.

G.8. How to record ICAE in the Case Card

In the Case Card (Appendix A) the entry about a counter-experience and ICAE is made in a constant form: what exactly happened, at which step of the micro-dynamics, which channels activated, what the durability is, what the next step is.

Example 1 (a fresh ICAE). Counter-experience: the client told something vulnerable and was not rejected. I level: I2 → I3 in the session. Channels: body — breathing changed, shoulders dropped; field — contact withstood; narrative — “I said it, and you didn’t turn away”; action — at work he once did not hide. Durability: L1, on the way to L2. Next step: repeatability without forcing; do not fix it in words more than necessary; do not turn a small experience into a plan.

Example 2 (oscillation, consolidation). Counter-experience: a small visibility without appraisal (a repetition after 3 weeks). I level: I2–I3, after a rollback to I1. Channels: body and field — stable; narrative — the client named it himself; action — two episodes outside the room. Durability: L2 (summoned deliberately under certain conditions). Signs of consolidation: the speed of return shortened from two weeks to a few days; breadth of transfer — close relationships; the power of the old RW lowered from RW3 to a stable RW2. Next step: hold the field, do not fix it as "achieved"; watch the rollbacks for their character, not for the fact itself.

Example 3 (a look-alike, not ICAE). Event: after an interpretation the client said "I understand, I need to learn to open up." I level: I0 (explanation). Channels: only narrative; no body, no field as lived, no action. Durability: none (an object of distinction, not an object of work as ICAE). Next step: do not fix the formulation; hear which minimal counter-experience would be fit for this form (M1–M2 from Appendix F); return to reading the Cα mode and the dominant constraint.

The entry is made in the language of the client's experience, not in the abstract language of the configuration. This holds the discipline: ICAE is something lived in the moment, not a category into which a session is filed.

End of Appendix G.

Appendix H. Atlas of 33 Phenomenological Invariants

A working support for Chapter 10. A map of phenomenological hearing: thirty-three forms of experience in eight groups.

H.1. How to use the atlas of invariants

This atlas unfolds what Chapter 10 names: thirty-three invariants — repeatable structural features of experience, grouped into eight functional groups. Each is given as a card for quick clinical hearing, not as an extended description. Before using it, one must hold several defenses:

- An invariant is not a symptom. A symptom says what manifests; an invariant, how experience is built from within.
- An invariant is not a diagnosis. It is a form of the organization of experience in the moment, not a category to which a person belongs.
- An invariant is not a theme. A theme says what is being talked about; an invariant, in what form of reality that talk becomes true.
- An invariant is a local structural feature. Not the whole organization of subjective reality, but one repeatable form of it.
- Invariants are read in clusters. A single invariant is rarely a complete formulation; what is clinically significant is the bundle of forms (see H.4 and Appendix I).
- A card helps one listen, it does not replace listening. To name an invariant is not to understand the person.

The main rule in reading the atlas: it is not a list of labels but a set of directions of hearing. Having heard one form, one asks which other forms hold beside it and what assembly they form together. The cards help formulate a hypothesis — not turn an invariant into a name for the client (more on the move from invariant to cluster in H.4).

Each card has six fields: structural definition, how to hear (speech, body, field, action), what to confuse it with, what is often premature, minimal counter-experience, frequent clusters. The "premature" and "counter-experience" fields are reading guides, not prescriptions: fit is always decided on the concrete material.

H.2. The eight groups of invariants

Eight directions of phenomenological hearing. The groups are navigation, not boxes: in a real person at a moment several forms from different groups are active, and they hold together.

- **Temporal (P-T1–P-T5).** Forms of time: whether the future is folded, whether the past lasts, whether the present has thinned, whether time stands still. Listen for what has happened to the temporal structure of experience.
- **World (P-W1–P-W4).** Forms of world: whether it is distanced, saturated with threat, has lost depth, whether the boundary between self and world has dissolved. Listen for what the world itself has become.
- **Self (P-SF1–P-SF4).** Forms of self-experience: whether the self is whole, distanced from experience, whether a coherent story of oneself holds, whether one is seized by shame, whether there is a stable witnessing support.
- **Salience (P-SA1–P-SA4).** Forms of what comes forward: the distribution of salience. What seizes attention against one's will, what matters, and whether the very capacity to give weight is intact.
- **Affective (P-AF1–P-AF4).** Forms of emotional tone: whether affect is available, what it is, whether it is experienced as one's own, whether there is safety, with what the experience is filled or emptied.
- **Intersubjective (P-IN1–P-IN4).** Forms of the other and the field: whether the other is present as alive, whether his gaze is dangerous, whether he holds, whether a shared common reality holds.
- **Agentic (P-AG1–P-AG4).** Forms of action and agency: whether action comes from me, whether "I can" is experienced, whether action is compelled, whether I observe it from the side.
- **Noetic (P-NO1–P-NO4).** Forms of meaning and directedness: whether meaning is present as density, whether the "what for" vector has collapsed, whether there is a calling and direction, whether there is a quality of the ultimate.

H.3. The thirty-three cards

— Temporal —

P-T1. Compression of the future. *Structural definition.* A form of time in which the future is folded to the almost-present: the distance between "now," "tomorrow," and "in a year" has collapsed, and no room is left in the future for anything to unfold. The future is neither empty nor taken away — it is compressed, and so is experienced as bearing down close, without air. Within this form the phrase "I have no future" is not a distortion but a precise description of a reality in which the future has truly lost its extension. *How to hear.* In speech — tomorrow and next year spoken of alike, without difference of scale; plans do not unfold, talk of "later" quickly folds back to "now." In the body — constriction, lack of air at the thought of the future. In the field — on being asked about plans, the very space of the conversation narrows, as if there is nowhere to put a plan. In action — "what's the point of guessing," a halt of forward-directed initiative. *What to confuse it with.* With depressive hopelessness as a theme — but here it is a form of time, not a mood about the future. With P-T5 (temporal standstill) — there the very flow of time stands still, here the extension of the future specifically is compressed. With a rupture of the self's link to the future — there the future as a category is whole but has no lived "I" in it; here the extension of the future itself is folded. *Often premature.* Planning, goal-setting, "small steps," reassurance "it will work out" — all require an unfolded future as a space, which is not there now. There is nowhere to put a plan, and non-fulfillment confirms the folding. *Minimal counter-experience.* A small experience that a gap has reappeared between "now" and "later": one experience in which the future unfolds by a step and time regains depth. Not a built plan but a sense of extension — that there is somewhere ahead to place even something. *Frequent clusters / where it occurs.* Often goes with the world compressed to the bearing-down (world), a halt of action (agentic), and an affect of no-way-out. Load-bearing invariant of CCP-1 (Compression of the future); occurs in the temporal-transitional family, sometimes beside P-T2 (intrusion of the past) under a general disorder of time.

P-T2. Intrusion of the past. *Structural definition.* A form of time in which the past has not passed: it lasts in the present as something happening now. "Then" is not closed and automatically organizes "now," so that the reaction in the present is clearly larger than the current event — the present is experienced through a long-ago scene. *How to hear.* In speech — disproportion of reaction to occasion, "as if it's happening again." In the body — reactions belonging to the former threat. In the field — today's other is met by the measure of a long-ago one. In action — behavior addressed to a past situation. The client may be aware of the mismatch and still react as then. *What to confuse it with.* With an actual conflict — but here the source of the reaction is in the past, not the present. With P-T1 — there the future is folded, here the past lasts. With P-AF (reactivated affect) — there the focus is the feeling, here the temporal structure: the very "when" has shifted. *Often premature.* Work only with the current event — it does not reach what organizes the reaction. Confrontation with the "irrationality" of the reaction strengthens the defense, because for the system the reaction is not irrational. *Minimal counter-experience.* A small experience of distinguishing "then" and "now": a moment in which the present is experienced as the present, not as a repetition. More often through the body and field than through explanation. *Frequent clusters / where it occurs.* Load-bearing invariant of CCP-2; temporal-transitional family. Often with developmental calibration and reactivated affect; sometimes with P-T1 under a general disorder of time.

P-T3. Thinning of the present. *Structural definition.* A form of time in which the present loses density: the moment is not lived but slips by, as if life is going on somewhere alongside and not here. Not a standstill of time and not its compression, but a loss of the saturation of the "now" itself — presence in the current moment thins. *How to hear.* In speech — "everything's in a fog," "I don't feel I'm living," difficulty recalling what filled the day. In the body — a muting of sensation. In the field — contact is there, but without involvement. In action — automatism, doing without presence. *What to confuse it with.* With P-W3 (flatness of the world) — there the world is bleached, here the time of the present is thinned. With dissociation as a symptom — the invariant describes a form, not a clinical category. With P-AF4 (emptying by grief) — there the emptiness is around a loss, here the density of the current moment is lost apart from any tie to loss. *Often premature.* Calls to "be here and now," intensification of experience — they require the saturation of the present that is not there now, and turn into pressure. *Minimal counter-experience.* A small experience of a filled instant: one sensation, sound, contact lived for a second as really present. A return of density, not a call to mindfulness. *Frequent clusters / where it occurs.* Temporal family; often beside P-W3 and blunted affect, sometimes in intersubjective absence (CCP-9), where the emptying of the field goes together with a thinning of presence.

P-T4. Predominance of the urgent future. *Structural definition.* A form of time in which the near future is experienced as a continuously bearing-down urgency: everything is on fire, everything must be managed in time, and the horizon is pulled tight to the next deadline. The far future may be intact but is screened off by the constant pressure of the nearest. *How to hear.* In speech — "no time," lists of the urgent, anxiety about being late. In the body — mobilization, inability to stop. In the field — hurriedness, difficulty withstanding the session's pause. In action — a race from urgent to urgent without respite. *What to confuse it with.* With P-T1 (compression of the future) — there the extension of the future in general is collapsed, here it is specifically the nearest that presses, while the far may be available. With P-AF1 (diffuse anxiety) — there anxiety without an object, here it is tied to the urgency of time. With thematic "busyness" — here it is a form of time, not a volume of tasks. *Often premature.* Time-management, prioritization — they require stepping out of the predominance of the urgent, which is itself what prevents applying them. Advice to "slow down" without an experience of a safe pause does not land. *Minimal counter-experience.* A small experience of a bearable pause: a moment in which stopping does not turn into catastrophe and the urgency lets go for a second. The experience that one can not run and the world does not collapse. *Frequent clusters / where it occurs.* Temporal family; often with diffuse anxiety and a mobilized body. May mask P-T1: beneath the race of the urgent the folding of the far future is sometimes hidden.

P-T5. Temporal standstill. *Structural definition.* A form of time in which its very flow has stopped: neither does the past recede, nor the future approach, time stands still. Often after a severe loss or trauma — the world froze at a point, and the movement of time does not resume. *How to hear.* In speech — "time stopped," "everything froze then." In the body — numbness, slowing. In the field — a sense of frozenness. In action — an impossibility of moving forward, life as if put on pause at a certain point. *What to confuse it with.* With P-T1 — there the future is compressed but time moves; here the very flow stands still. With P-T2 — there the past actively intrudes; here movement has frozen, the past not so much intruding as not letting go by holding. With depressive retardation as a symptom — the invariant is about a form of time, not a clinical category. *Often premature.* Urging to "move on," an orientation to the future — they require a resumed flow of time, which is not there, and sound like a failure to understand the standstill. *Minimal counter-experience.* A small experience of resumed movement: an experience in which time takes one step — something after the point of the standstill is felt for the first time as "later," not as a frozen "then." *Frequent clusters / where it occurs.* Temporal-transitional family; often with emptying by grief (P-AF4) and a thinning of the present. May be load-bearing in frozen transition (CCP-10), where the standstill of time joins with supportlessness.

— World —

P-W1. Distance of the world. *Structural definition.* A form of world in which it is distanced: perceived as if through glass or a film, not reaching, not touching. The world is there, but at a remove, and between the person and the world is a layer through which nothing passes fully. *How to hear.* In speech — "as if behind glass," "everything's far away," "it doesn't reach me." In the body — a muting of perception. In the field — contact goes through a distance. In action — involvement without full touch of the world. *What to confuse it with.* With P-W3 (flatness of the world) — there the world lost depth and salience, here it is preserved but distanced. With P-IN3 (intersubjective absence) — there it is specifically the other that became lifeless, here the world as a whole is distanced. With derealization as a symptom — the invariant is about a form, not a label. *Often premature.* Intensification of contact with the world, sensory tasks "feel this" — they require a nearness of the world that is not there now, and run into the distance. *Minimal counter-experience.* A small experience of touch: one moment in which the world reaches for a second — a sound, light, a touch that passed through the film. A return of nearness in a small dose. *Frequent clusters / where it occurs.* World family; often with a thinning of the present and blunted affect. Neighbors self-distance (P-SF1), when both the world and one's own experience are distanced.

P-W2. Threat-saturation of the world. *Structural definition.* A form of world in which it is steeped in threat: the environment is read as dangerous as a whole, not at a particular point. Not a single fear, but a background quality of the world — it is unfriendly, and at any moment misfortune may come. *How to hear.* In speech — "the world is dangerous," wariness toward the environment, expectation of the bad. In the body — chronic readiness, scanning. In the field — distrust of the room's safety. In action — defensive avoidance, checking the exits. *What to confuse it with.* With P-SA2 (threat-capture of attention) — there attention is pulled to threat as a focus of salience, here threat is diffused as a quality of the world itself. With P-AF1 (diffuse anxiety) — there affect without an object, here a form of the world as threatening. With a real danger of the environment (Λ) — important to check: if the world objectively produces threat, protection comes first, not reading the form. *Often premature.* Cognitive disputation of danger, "the world isn't so frightening" — arguing with content is useless while threat holds as a form of the world; exposure without safety of the field is premature. *Minimal counter-experience.* A small experience of a safe patch of world: a moment or place experienced as non-threatening — that at least here and now the world is not attacking. *Frequent clusters / where it occurs.* World family; often with diffuse anxiety, a scanning body, sometimes with aberrant salience (P-SA3) at a shift toward O4–O5. Check Λ before reading it as an inner form.

P-W3. Flatness of the world. *Structural definition.* A form of world in which it has lost depth and relief: everything is one tone, nothing stands out, the world is bleached and flat. Not threat and not distance, but a loss of the dimension of salience in the world itself — it has become even and dull. *How to hear.* In speech — "everything's gray," "nothing catches," "I don't care." In the body — sluggishness, absence of response. In the field — evenness without animation. In action — absence of any pull toward anything in the world. *What to confuse it with.* With P-SA1 (global loss of salience) — close, but P-W3 is about a form of the world (it is flat), P-SA1 about the distribution of salience (nothing comes forward); they often go together. With P-AF (blunting of affect) — there the focus is emotional tone, here the quality of the world. With P-NO2 (collapse of meaning) — there the "what for" directedness has collapsed, here the world itself is bleached. *Often premature.* Urging toward interest, searching for "what used to gladden you" — they require a relief of the world that is not there; reassurance bounces off the flatness. *Minimal counter-experience.* A small experience of relief: one moment in which something in the world slightly stands out — a color, a taste, a detail that for a second stopped being gray. *Frequent clusters / where it occurs.* World family; tightly with P-SA1 and blunted affect. A frequent support of depressive assemblies; may neighbor a global loss of meaning.

P-W4. Permeability / dissolution of the world. *Structural definition.* A form of world in which the boundaries between self and world thin: the outer penetrates inward, the inner outward, separateness is lost. In a marked form the world and self lose a clear boundary, and the experience of protected separateness collapses. This is a risky form, requiring a reading of the O vertical. *How to hear.* In speech — "everything penetrates," "no protection," "can't separate myself from what's happening." In the body — absence of a boundary, unprotectedness. In the field — merging with the state of the other. In action — being seized by the external without a filter. Hear the degree: from heightened impressionability to a loss of the self–world boundary. *What to confuse it with.* With P-W1 (distance of the world) — the direct opposite: there the world is distanced, here the boundary is dissolved. With a disturbance of P-IN1 (the field of shared reality) — close at a shift up the O axis. With empathic sensitivity — there the boundary is intact and restorable, here it is lost. *Often premature.* Opening, regressive, depth interventions — they strengthen the dissolution of the boundary; work toward "greater openness to the world" is contraindicated while the boundary is unstable. *Minimal counter-experience.* A small experience of a restored boundary: a moment in which protected separateness is experienced — that between me and the world there is skin again. Support, contour, grounding. *Frequent clusters / where it occurs.* World family; at a shift toward O4–O5 it joins with a disturbance of the field of shared reality and aberrant salience. Boundary of safety: at a loss of reality testing, specialized assessment comes first, not work with the form.

— Self —

P-SF1. Self-distance. *Structural definition.* A form of self-experience in which the person is distanced from his own experience: he observes himself from the side, as a stranger, and does not live what is happening as his own. Not an absence of self, but a split between the experiencing and the experienced — the "I" looks at the "I" from afar. *How to hear.* In speech — "as if it's not happening to me," "I watch myself from the side," telling of oneself in the third plane. In the body — estrangement from sensation. In the field — presence without involvement of the self. In action — doing without experiencing authorship of the experience. *What to confuse it with.* With P-SF4 (witnessing "I") — an important distinction: P-SF1 is an estranged split (I observe myself as a stranger), P-SF4 is an integrative form (there is a stable witnessing support without loss of self). With P-W1 — there the world is distanced, here one's own experience. With dissociation as a symptom — the invariant is about a form, not a category. *Often premature.* Deepening into experience, "stay with the feeling" — they require presence in the experience from which there is now a distance; pressing strengthens the withdrawal. *Minimal counter-experience.* A small experience of presence in oneself: a moment in which experience is felt as one's own, from within, not observed from the side. A brief return into one's own experience. *Frequent clusters / where it occurs.* Self family; often with distance of the world and a thinning of the present. When marked and with unstable coherence — read the O vertical.

P-SF2. Collapse of the narrative "I". *Structural definition.* A form of self-experience in which the coherent story of oneself breaks down: the "I" does not hold as a character continuing through time, the biography falls into disconnected pieces. Not the particular content of the story, but the very capacity to assemble oneself into a coherent narrative. *How to hear.* In speech — contradictory, unstitchable versions of oneself, "I don't know who I am," breaks in the biographical thread. In the body — heterogeneity of states. In the field — different "I"s from session to session. In action — inconsistency not explained by circumstances. *What to confuse it with.* With P-SF1 (self-distance) — there the "I" is whole but distanced; here the coherence of the story itself falls apart. With P-SF3 (globalization of the shame-"I") — there the "I" is assembled around a defect (too coherently and negatively), here it does not assemble at all. With ordinary contradictoriness — here it is specifically the impossibility of narrative assembly, not a richness of facets. *Often premature.* Work on the "real I," integrative narrative tasks — they require the support of a coherent "I" that is not there; premature under an unstable assembly. *Minimal counter-experience.* A small experience of the thread: a moment in which two pieces of oneself link into one lived line — "it was, after all, me." A return of minimal continuity. *Frequent clusters / where it occurs.* Self family; when marked, linked with dissociative fragmentation — read the O vertical (often O4). May neighbor frozen transition (CCP-10).

P-SF3. Globalization of the shame-"I". *Structural definition.* A form of self-experience in which shame seizes the whole "I": not "I did something bad," but "I am, entirely, a defect." Shame stops being a reaction to a deed and becomes a total quality of the self — the "I" as a whole is read as shameful. *How to hear.* In speech — "there's something wrong with me in principle," "I'm just bad," a generalization of the single to the total. In the body — contraction, a wish to vanish. In the field — expectation of total condemnation. In action — hiding oneself as a whole, not a separate deed. *What to confuse it with.* With P-AF2 (shame collapse) — an important distinction: P-AF2 is an affective form (an overwhelming feeling of shame), P-SF3 is a self form (the structure "I am, entirely, a defect"); they often go together, but these are different layers. With P-IN2 (threat of being seen) — there an intersubjective form (the other's gaze is dangerous), here a self form (I am shameful in and of myself). With CCP-4 — that is a configuration holding the shame reality by a bundle of invariants; P-SF3 is one of its load-bearing ones, not the whole assembly. *Often premature.* Direct disputation "you're not bad," praise — they strengthen the exposure of the shameful "I" and are read as one more appraisal; work with a particular deed does not reach the totality. *Minimal counter-experience.* A small experience of partiality: a moment in which something separate, not "all of me," turns out to be shameful — and one remains accepted nonetheless. A return of the boundary between deed and self. *Frequent clusters / where it occurs.* Self family; load-bearing invariant of CCP-4 together with P-IN2 and P-AF2. Often with the threat of being seen and shame collapse; self-protective family.

P-SF4. Emergence of the witnessing "I". *Structural definition.* A form of self-experience in which a stable observing support appears: an "I" that can be present at its own experience without merging with it and without losing itself. An integrative form — not detachment, but a gained capacity to be a witness of one's experience while remaining within it. *How to hear.* In speech — "I noticed this rising in me," describing experience from a stable point of observation without estrangement. In the body — support, centeredness. In the field — an ability to reflect on the process as it goes. In action — a pause of observation between impulse and reaction. *What to confuse it with.* With P-SF1 (self-distance) — critical not to confuse: P-SF1 is an estranged split from experience, P-SF4 a present witnessing without loss of self. With intellectualization — there a flight from experience into thought, here contact with experience is preserved alongside observation. *Often premature.* This is an integrative form — what is premature is not to "evoke" it but to load it with expectation: to demand reflection where there is not yet support, or to turn witnessing into a technique of self-control. *Minimal counter-experience.* Here the invariant is itself the form the counter-experience strengthens: to help the witnessing "I" take hold — to resonate in the body, to sound in contact, to find a word — so that it gains a path to repetition. Not to produce reflection, but to let the support grow firm. *Frequent clusters / where it occurs.* Self family; an integrative marker. Often appears together with restored agency (P-AG3) and the presence of meaning (P-NO1) as a sign of a growing stability of the assembly.

— Salience —

P-SA1. Global loss of salience. *Structural definition.* A form of salience in which the field of experience loses salience as a whole: nothing comes forward, nothing is more important than anything else, salience is zeroed. This is a loss of the very distribution of importance — not "what is more important," but that nothing at all stands out as salient. *How to hear.* In speech — "I don't care," "nothing matters," an inability to prefer. In the body — absence of pull, inertness. In the field — even indifference. In action — absence of motivation, because nothing is singled out as worth it. *What to confuse it with.* With P-NO2 (collapse of meaning) — a key pair: P-SA1 is about salience (what comes forward in the field of experience — nothing), P-NO2 about meaning-directedness (the "what for," the vector of life, has collapsed). Salience answers "what matters now," meaning "toward what is it directed." They often go together, but these are different axes. With P-W3 (flatness of the world) — there the world is bleached, here the distribution of salience is zeroed. *Often premature.* A search for goals, "what's important to you" — they require a working distribution of salience that is not there; the question hangs in indifference. *Minimal counter-experience.* A small experience of standing-out: a moment in which one thing slightly comes forward as a bit more important — a return of the very capacity to give weight. *Frequent clusters / where it occurs.* Salience family; tightly with flatness of the world and blunted affect, often beside the collapse of meaning (P-NO2). A support of depressive and anhedonic assemblies.

P-SA2. Threat-capture of attention. *Structural definition.* A form of salience in which salience is pulled to threat: attention is automatically captured by the dangerous, and everything else loses weight. The logic of distributing salience is intact but skewed — threat draws the whole field of the important onto itself. *How to hear.* In speech — a return to the dangerous, difficulty holding attention on the neutral. In the body — scanning, flinching. In the field — hypervigilance to signals of disapproval or danger. In action — the priority of defense over everything else. *What to confuse it with.* With P-W2 (threat-saturation of the world) — there threat is diffused as a quality of the world, here pulled in as a focus of attention. With P-SA3 (aberrant salience) — there the very distribution is disturbed (the neutral becomes addressed), here the distribution is intact but shifted toward threat. With P-AF1 (diffuse anxiety) — there affect without an object, here attention tied to threat. *Often premature.* Switching attention "look at the good," positive reorientation — they do not land while threat holds the salience; they require first a lowering of the capture. *Minimal counter-experience.* A small experience of a shift of focus: a moment in which attention lets go of the threat for a second and is held on the neutral or safe without anxiety. *Frequent clusters / where it occurs.* Salience family; often with threat-saturation of the world, diffuse anxiety, a scanning body. A frequent support of anxious and post-traumatic assemblies.

P-SA3. Aberrant salience. *Structural definition.* A form of salience in which salience is distributed not by the usual logic of the relevant: what would normally stay background becomes salient, and connections between events are experienced as loaded with a special meaning against one's will. This is not a richness of associations but a failure of the very distribution of importance — when the neutral comes forward as personally addressed, and the ordinary filter of the salient stops holding. In a marked form aberrant salience begins to organize experienced reality. *How to hear.* In speech — a special significance of random details, coincidences, signs; a sense that what is happening is addressed, although there is no addressing. In affect — a tense captivation, sometimes anxiety or elevation around the "significant." In the field — difficulty returning details to a neutral background. Important to hear the degree: from a heightened sensitivity to meanings to experiences that organize reality against any check. *What to confuse it with.* With P-SA2 (threat-capture of attention) — there salience is pulled to danger, but the logic of the relevant is intact; here the distribution itself is disturbed. With intellectual liveliness and a leaning toward interpretation — but there connections are checkable and releasable, here the loadedness does not let go. With noetic overload (CCP-8) — there everything is significant at once from an excess of meaning, but without a failure of reality testing; aberrant salience may be its edge at a shift toward O4–O5. *Often premature.* Deepening of meanings, joint search for "what this means," work with the content of the signs — all this adds salience instead of lowering the load. And before any such work: at signs that salience is beginning to organize reality against any check, what comes first is not phenomenological work but an assessment of the stability of the assembly. *Minimal counter-experience.* A small experience of the neutral: a moment in which a detail can stay simply background, unaddressed and unloaded. A rest from salience, a support on the ordinary and on the reality-check shared with another — not a new meaning. *Frequent clusters / where it occurs.* Neighbors threat-saturation of the world (P-W2), a tense affect, and sometimes permeability of the world (P-W4). May be a load-bearing edge of CCP-8 at a shift toward O4–O5. Boundary of safety: with a disturbance of reality testing this is not an object of work with the configuration but a ground for specialized assessment — safety is engaged because the current assembly shows a risk of disorganization, not because this invariant has been named.

P-SA4. Predominance of social signals. *Structural definition.* A form of salience in which salience is pulled to social signals: the looks, tone, expressions, approval and disapproval of others draw the whole field of the important onto themselves. Social appraisal becomes the main thing that comes forward, and screens off the rest. *How to hear.* In speech — a constant reference to what others will think, how it was received. In the body — a tuning to the other's reaction. In the field — an over-sensitivity to the slightest signal from the therapist. In action — behavior led by an expected appraisal. *What to confuse it with.* With P-IN2 (threat of being seen) — there an intersubjective form (visibility is dangerous), here a salience one (social signals pull the salience). With P-SF3 (globalization of the shame-"I") — there a self structure, here a distribution of attention. With ordinary social sensitivity — here it is specifically a predominance that screens off the rest. *Often premature.* Advice to "pay no attention to others," work toward autonomy of appraisal — they require a redistribution of salience that is not there; they do not land while the social holds the weight. *Minimal counter-experience.* A small experience of non-social salience: a moment in which something matters in itself, apart from another's appraisal — a return of weight to what is not about the other's gaze. *Frequent clusters / where it occurs.* Salience family; often with the threat of being seen (P-IN2) and shame forms. A frequent companion of the shame organization (CCP-4) and of attachment without differentiation (CCP-5).

— Affective —

P-AF1. Diffuse anxiety. *Structural definition.* A form of affect in which anxiety is present without an object: a background tension not tied to a concrete threat. Not a fear of something, but an anxious tone of existence itself — body and psyche in readiness, but it is unclear toward what. *How to hear.* In speech — "anxious, but I don't know why," objectless unease. In the body — tension, restlessness, shallow breathing. In the field — a background tension without a clear cause. In action — restless activity without direction. *What to confuse it with.* With P-SA2 (threat-capture of attention) — there is an object-threat holding attention; here anxiety is objectless. With P-W2 (threat-saturation of the world) — there the world is read as dangerous, here there is not even an image of danger. With P-T4 (predominance of the urgent) — there anxiety is tied to the urgency of time, here it is objectless. *Often premature.* A search for "what you're anxious about," cognitive work with content — they run into the objectlessness; demanding to name the cause strengthens the anxiety. *Minimal counter-experience.* A small experience of regulation without explanation: a moment in which the body calms — breath, grounding, field — and the anxious tone lets go without the need to find a cause. *Frequent clusters / where it occurs.* Affective family; often with a mobilized body, threat-saturation of the world, predominance of the urgent. A support of generalized-anxious assemblies.

P-AF2. Shame collapse. *Structural definition.* A form of affect in which shame overwhelms entirely: not a signal emotion but a crashing wave under which coherence falls. An affective experience of shame of such force that the system does not hold it and contracts, falls through, vanishes. *How to hear.* In speech — a break, falling silent, "I want to sink through the floor." In the body — contraction, heat, averting the gaze, a wish to disappear. In the field — a sudden closing-down at the touch of the shameful. In action — withdrawal, cessation of contact. *What to confuse it with.* With P-SF3 (globalization of the shame-"I") — the key pair: P-AF2 is an affective wave (the feeling overwhelms), P-SF3 a self structure ("I am, entirely, a defect"); often together, but different layers. With P-IN2 (threat of being seen) — there an intersubjective form (the gaze is dangerous), here an affective collapse. With ordinary shame as a reaction — here it is specifically a collapse of coherence under affect. *Often premature.* Naming the shame at the moment of the crash, deepening — they strengthen the overwhelm and provoke withdrawal; work with shame is premature while there is no stability of the field. *Minimal counter-experience.* A small experience of held shame: a moment in which shame rose but coherence did not crash and contact was preserved — that shame can be lived through without vanishing. *Frequent clusters / where it occurs.* Affective family; load-bearing in CCP-4 together with P-SF3 and P-IN2. Self-protective family; when coherence falls at the touch — read the thresholds Θ.

P-AF3. Softening into safety. *Structural definition.* A form of affect in which a lived safety appears: body and field let go, readiness gives way to calm, it becomes possible not to defend. An integrative form — not an absence of anxiety, but an active experience that one can be safe now.

How to hear. In speech — "it's calm here," "I can exhale." In the body — relaxation of the shoulders, deepening of breath, support. In the field — a lowering of wariness, trust in contact. In action — giving up defensive movements, openness. *What to confuse it with.* With a mere absence of an anxiety-stimulus — here an active experience of safety, not a temporary lull. With a compliant "all is well" — there an adjustment, here a bodily-lived calm. With P-AF4 (emptying) — there emptiness, here a filled calm. *Often premature.* This is an integrative form — what is premature is to load it: to bring in difficult material at once "now that it's calm," or to declare safety achieved. A fragile calm is easily startled by load. *Minimal counter-experience.* Here the invariant is itself the form the counter-experience strengthens: to help the softening into safety take hold — to resonate in the body, to sound in contact, to find a word — so that it gains a path to repetition. To let the calm grow firm, without hurrying it. *Frequent clusters / where it occurs.* Affective family; an integrative support on which other counter-experiences become possible. Often precedes restored agency (P-AG3) and attuned holding (P-IN4).

P-AF4. Emptying by grief. *Structural definition.* A form of affect in which grief leaves an emptiness: after a loss the world and self are emptied, in place of the former fullness — a void. Not acute pain, but the emptiness of loss — what was filled by a presence has become hollow. *How to hear.* In speech — "empty inside," "everything has emptied out," speech about the absence of what was. In the body — heaviness, depletion. In the field — the presence of the loss in contact. In action — a meaninglessness of what used to be done for or with the lost one. *What to confuse it with.* With P-W3 (flatness of the world) — there the world is flat without a tie to loss, here the emptiness is around a particular loss. With P-SA1 (loss of salience) — there the distribution of importance in general is zeroed, here an emptying from a loss. With P-T5 (temporal standstill) — often together, but P-T5 is about time, P-AF4 about an affect of emptiness. *Often premature.* Urging to "move on," filling the void with the new — premature: the emptiness of grief requires first that one be able to withstand it, not close it. *Minimal counter-experience.* A small experience of a bearable emptiness: a moment in which the emptiness of grief is experienced and held in the presence of another, without requiring filling. That the void can be withstood not alone. *Frequent clusters / where it occurs.* Affective family; often with temporal standstill (P-T5) and a thinning of the present. A support of grieving assemblies; a self-standing form of loss.

— Intersubjective —

P-IN1. Field of shared reality. *Structural definition.* A form of intersubjectivity in which a field of shared common reality holds with another: we are with the other in one world, meanings coincide, reality is confirmed in the meeting. A basic integrative form — its disturbance is read along the O vertical as a risk of disorganization. *How to hear.* In speech — a natural reliance on common understanding, a coincidence of meanings without checking. In the body — co-attunement. In the field — an experience of a common space of meaning. The disturbance is heard as a falling-out of shared reality: meanings stop coinciding, the sharedness of the field tears. *What to confuse it with.* With P-IN4 (attuned holding) — P-IN1 is about the basic sharedness of reality, P-IN4 about precise affective co-attunement within it. With P-W4 (dissolution of the world) — at a disturbance they join: the loss of boundary and the loss of shared reality go together at a shift toward O4–O5. With ordinary agreement — here it is the very fabric of shared reality, not a coincidence of opinions. *Often premature.* At a disturbance of shared reality any work with content is premature — an assessment of the stability of the assembly comes first; when intact, it is a background, not a target. *Minimal counter-experience.* A small experience of restored sharedness: a moment in which there is again one field of reality with another, meanings coincide, and this is experienced as a support. *Frequent clusters / where it occurs.* Intersubjective family; an integrative base. The disturbance — at a shift toward O4–O5, beside permeability of the world and aberrant salience. Boundary of safety: with a disturbance of reality testing, specialized assessment comes first.

P-IN2. Threat of being seen. *Structural definition.* A form of intersubjectivity in which visibility is experienced as a threat: to be seen means to be exposed to condemnation. The other's gaze is dangerous in itself — not for something particular, but as an exposure under which one is destroyed. *How to hear.* In speech — a fear of attention, a wish not to stand out, apologies for one's presence. In the body — contraction under a gaze, averting the eyes. In the field — wariness toward the therapist's appraisal, reading a neutral face as condemning. In action — a dosed presenting of oneself, checking the reaction. *What to confuse it with.* With P-SF3 (globalization of the shame-"I") — there a self structure ("I am, entirely, a defect"), here an intersubjective one (the other's gaze is dangerous); often together. With P-SA4 (predominance of social signals) — there salience is pulled to the social, here it is specifically visibility that is experienced as a threat. With

CCP-4 — that is a configuration; P-IN2 is one of its load-bearing invariants, not the whole assembly. *Often premature.* Direct naming of shame, praise, exposure tasks "present yourself" — they strengthen the threat of visibility while the field is not yet lived as safe for it. *Minimal counter-experience.* A small experience of visibility without appraisal: a moment in which the client is seen — and not judged, not comforted too quickly, not corrected. That here one can be seen and not be destroyed. *Frequent clusters / where it occurs.* Intersubjective family; load-bearing in CCP-4 together with P-SF3 and P-AF2. Often with predominance of social signals; a self-protective assembly.

P-IN3. Intersubjective absence. *Structural definition.* A form of intersubjectivity in which the other is not present as alive: the field has emptied of people, they are there physically but are not experienced as real presences. Contact goes through glass — not loneliness as a feeling, but a loss of the liveness of the other. *How to hear.* In speech — describing relationships without liveness, "as if behind glass." In the body — absence of co-attunement. In the field — contact does not form despite formal correctness; the therapist may feel invisible or interchangeable. In action — functional interaction without a meeting. *What to confuse it with.* With P-W1 (distance of the world) — there the world as a whole is distanced, here it is specifically the other that became lifeless. With attachment without differentiation (CCP-5) — the opposite: there the other is too much, to the point of merging, here he is not there at all. With introverted reserve — here it is specifically a loss of the liveness of the other, not a preference. *Often premature.* Calls to closeness "let's stay in contact," emotionally saturated interventions — the field does not withstand a living presence, and pressing strengthens the withdrawal behind glass. *Minimal counter-experience.* A small experience of a living presence in a small dose: a brief moment in which the other is experienced as real and this is bearable. A dose of liveness the field is able to let through. *Frequent clusters / where it occurs.* Intersubjective family; load-bearing in CCP-9. Often with blunted affect, a thinning of the present, self-distance; with marked dissociation — read the O vertical.

P-IN4. Attuned holding. *Structural definition.* A form of intersubjectivity in which the other holds by a precise co-attunement: present, responsive, holding — without merging and without withdrawing. An integrative form of the field, in which one experiences being precisely felt and held. *How to hear.* In speech — "you understood," "here I am held." In the body — co-attunement, a response to the response. In the field — an experience of precise holding, the rhythm of the meeting. In action — reliance on the other's presence without merging with it. *What to confuse it with.* With P-IN1 (field of shared reality) — P-IN4 is about precise affective co-attunement, P-IN1 about the basic sharedness of reality. With attachment without differentiation (CCP-5) — there holding is needed to the point of inseparability, here it supports separateness. With a mere alliance — here it is specifically a lived precise holding, not a working agreement. *Often premature.* This is an integrative form — what is premature is to exploit it: to bring in the difficult at once "now that there's contact," or to turn holding into an instrument of pressure. *Minimal counter-experience.* Here the invariant is itself the form the counter-experience strengthens: to help the attuned holding take hold — to resonate in the body, to sound in contact, to find a word — so that it becomes a support one can return to. *Frequent clusters / where it occurs.* Intersubjective family; an integrative base on which other counter-experiences become possible. Often precedes the counter-experience of visibility without appraisal (in work with CCP-4) and restored agency.

— Agentic —

P-AG1. Impossibility of action. *Structural definition.* A form of agency in which action is unavailable: "I can" has vanished, between intention and action there is a void, and movement does not begin. Not unwillingness, but an absence of the very experience of available outgoing action. *How to hear.* In speech — "I can't make myself," "it doesn't get done by itself," describing life in the passive voice. In the body — numbness, heaviness, an inability to initiate. In the field — an expectation that movement will come from outside. In action — a paralysis of initiative. *What to confuse it with.* With P-AG4 (observer without agency) — the key pair: P-AG1 — action is unavailable at all, P-AG4 — the subject acts or could, but observes himself, not experiencing himself as the source. With laziness or resistance as a theme — here it is specifically a loss of the experience of "I can." With P-AG2 (compelled action) — there action exists but is compelled; here it does not exist. *Often premature.* Activating tasks, "start small," plans — they require an agency that is not there; non-fulfillment confirms the powerlessness. Check the body and the environment, where the veto more often holds. *Minimal counter-experience.* A small experience of outgoing action: a micro-movement experienced as "I did this" — a return of authorship in the smallest thing, not a result. *Frequent clusters / where it occurs.* Agentic family; load-bearing in CCP-6. Often with bodily exhaustion, emptying, collapse of meaning; check B(t) and Λ as frequent veto layers.

P-AG2. Compelled action. *Structural definition.* A form of agency in which action exists but is experienced as compelled: not one's own, imposed from within or without, carried out without authorship. "I do," but not "I want" — action is estranged from the subject while the capacity to act is intact. *How to hear.* In speech — "I have to," "I must," "I can't not," action under the pressure of duty or compulsion. In the body — the tension of execution without pull. In the field — performing the expected. In action — activity without an experienced choice. *What to confuse it with.* With P-AG1 (impossibility of action) — there action is unavailable, here it exists but compelled. With P-AG3 (restored agency) — the direct opposite: there authorship has returned, here it is absent though action exists. With compulsion as a symptom — the invariant is about a form of the experience of authorship, not a category. *Often premature.* Urging toward greater activity, loading with responsibility — they add compulsion; work on "do what you must" strengthens the estrangement of action. *Minimal counter-experience.* A small experience of chosen action: a moment in which even something small is done out of "I want," not "I must" — a return of the experience of authorship in action. *Frequent clusters / where it occurs.* Agentic family; often beside collapse of agency (CCP-6) as its neighbor and with a predominance of duty. May masquerade as productivity in the absence of authorship.

P-AG3. Restored agency. *Structural definition.* A form of action in which the experience of "I can" returns: action again comes from the subject, not only happens to him. This is not an achievement and not a result, but a return of authorship — the moment when the experienced link between intention and action is restored and the person again feels himself the source of even the smallest movement. An integrative form: it is heard not as a "good state" but as a structural shift in where action comes from. *How to hear.* In speech — a move from the passive voice to the active: "I decided," "I did it myself" instead of "it doesn't get done by itself." In the body — support, straightening, an initiating movement. In the field — the client leads a little more, waits for permission a little less. Often it sounds quiet and in passing — like "I may not come close," said for the first time as a new possibility, not as a report. *What to confuse it with.* With an elevated mood or a compliant "I'm doing fine" — but there is no experience of outgoing action there, only affect or adjustment. With compelled action (P-AG2) —

there action exists but is experienced as compelled, not one's own; here it is specifically authorship that has returned. With discharge (CCP-7) — there action bypasses meaning; here it passes through the subject. *Often premature.* Loading restored agency with more weight than it holds: praise, "see, you can," expansion into plans and obligations. An early form of agency is fragile; loaded with expectation, it easily returns to collapse. It is also premature to hurry repetition while the experience has not taken hold in several channels. *Minimal counter-experience.* Here the invariant is itself the form the counter-experience strengthens: to help restored agency resonate in the body, sound in contact, find a word, and link to a possible next small action — so that it gains a path to repetition. To hold the moment without loading it, rather than declaring victory. *Frequent clusters / where it occurs.* Often appears as a shift within the agentic-active family — the first sign of emerging from the collapse of agency (CCP-6) or from compelled action. Goes together with the return of the vector (noetic forms) and a revival of affect. Clinically — a frequent marker that the accumulation of minimal counter-experiences has begun to shift the reality weight of the old configuration.

P-AG4. Observer without agency. *Structural definition.* A form of agency in which the subject observes his own action without experiencing himself as its source: action occurs, but the "I" looks at it from the side, as at a stranger's. Not an absence of action, but a split between the acting and the observing. *How to hear.* In speech — "I watched myself do it," "as if it wasn't I who acted." In the body — estrangement from one's own movements. In the field — presence without authorship. In action — deeds experienced as observed, not performed. *What to confuse it with.* With P-AG1 (impossibility of action) — there action is unavailable, here it exists but without the experience of authorship. With P-SF1 (self-distance) — close, but P-SF1 is about self-experience as a whole, P-AG4 specifically about the source of action. With dissociation as a symptom — the invariant is about a form, not a label. *Often premature.* Placing responsibility for the actions, "you did it yourself" — they run into the rupture of authorship; demanding to own the action is premature while the rupture holds. *Minimal counter-experience.* A small experience of owned action: a moment in which action is experienced as coming from the "I," not observed from the side — a joining of the observing and the acting. *Frequent clusters / where it occurs.* Agentic family; when marked — read the O vertical (often dissociative fragmentation). Neighbors self-distance (P-SF1) and the collapse of the narrative "I".

— Noetic —

P-NO1. Presence of meaning. *Structural definition.* A form of meaning in which it is present as density and coherence: life holds as meaningful, events are connected, there is a "for the sake of which." An integrative noetic form — not the particular content of meaning, but its presence as a support. *How to hear.* In speech — a natural coherence of "what for" and "for the sake of," a semantic density of the telling. In the body — collectedness, the tone of directedness. In the field — a shared experience of the meaningful. In action — actions linked by a common meaning. *What to confuse it with.* With P-NO4 (vocation / directedness) — P-NO1 is about the presence of meaning as density and coherence, P-NO4 about its vector, calling, directedness toward something. With an elevated mood — there affect, here a semantic support. With P-SA presence of salience — there what comes forward, here what it is lived for. *Often premature.* This is an integrative form — what is premature is to load it with a demand for more meaning or turn it into an obligation to "find meaning." *Minimal counter-experience.* Here the invariant is itself the form the counter-experience strengthens: to help the presence of meaning take hold — to resonate in the body, to sound in contact, to find a word, to link with action — so that it gains a path to repetition. *Frequent clusters / where it occurs.* Noetic family; an integrative support. Often appears with restored agency (P-AG3) and the witnessing "I" (P-SF4) as a sign of growing stability.

P-NO2. Collapse of meaning. *Structural definition.* A form of meaning in which directedness has collapsed: the "what for" has fallen, the vector of life has vanished, nothing leads. Not a loss of salience (what comes forward), but a collapse of meaning itself — there is no "for the sake of which," and the directedness of existence has fallen apart. *How to hear.* In speech — "everything's meaningless," "what's all this for," a loss of the "for the sake of." In the body — a slackening, a loss of the tone of directedness. In the field — the absence of a projected future meaning. In action — a halt of what was held by meaning. *What to confuse it with.* With P-SA1 (global loss of salience) — the key pair: P-NO2 is about meaning-directedness (the "what for" has fallen), P-SA1 about salience (nothing comes forward). One can lose the vector while keeping the capacity to give weight, and vice versa; often together. With P-W3 (flatness of the world) — there the world is bleached, here meaning has collapsed. *Often premature.* A search for meaning "what is there for you to live for," existential tasks — they require a support of directedness that is not there; premature while meaning has collapsed. *Minimal counter-experience.* A small experience of a small directedness: a moment in which at least some "for the sake of" appears — even a small movement toward something, returning the vector. *Frequent clusters / where it occurs.* Noetic family; often with a global loss of salience (P-SA1) and flatness of the world. A support of existential-depressive assemblies.

P-NO3. Sacred quality. *Structural definition.* A form of meaning in which something is experienced as possessing a special quality exceeding the ordinary — sacred, ultimate, absolutely significant. In a moderate form — a support and depth; at a shift toward O4–O5 it may join with aberrant salience and require a reading of the O vertical. *How to hear.* In speech — an experience of the ultimate, the holy, the absolute importance of something. In the body — awe, trembling. In the field — a special quality of the significant. In action — devotion to what is experienced as sacred. Hear the degree: from a supportive depth to a captivation that organizes reality. *What to confuse it with.* With P-NO4 (vocation) — there a vector-directedness, here a quality of ultimate significance. With P-SA3 (aberrant salience) — at a shift toward O4–O5 they join: the sacred quality may become aberrant. With cultural-religious experience — important not to pathologize: in its context this is an intact form; read the degree and the stability of the assembly, not the content. *Often premature.* Disputation or interpretation of the sacred, the reduction "really this is about…" — they destroy the support and do not land. At a shift toward O4–O5 an assessment of stability comes first, not work with the content. *Minimal counter-experience.* When the form is supportive, it need not be shifted — it is held as a resource. A counter-experience is appropriate at the neighboring forms; here what matters more is to distinguish the supportive sacred from the aberrant along the O vertical. *Frequent clusters / where it occurs.* Noetic family; in its supportive form — beside the presence of meaning and directedness. At a shift toward O4–O5 — beside aberrant salience; the boundary of safety by reality testing, read contextually and culturally.

P-NO4. Vocation / directedness. *Structural definition.* A form of meaning in which it has a vector: there is a calling, a directedness toward something, a pull leading forward. An integrative noetic form — not simply the presence of meaning, but its aspiration, the experience of "where to" and "for the sake of what, forward." *How to hear.* In speech — "I'm drawn to…," "I know what for," an experience of a calling and a direction. In the body — aspiration, the tone of forward movement. In the field — a shared experience of directedness. In action — actions built by a vector. *What to* *confuse it with.* With P-NO1 (presence of meaning) — P-NO4 is about the vector and the calling, P-NO1 about the density and coherence of meaning; directedness presupposes presence but adds aspiration. With P-T future — there a form of time, here a semantic vector. With ambition — there a goal-achievement, here a lived calling. *Often premature.* This is an integrative form — what is premature is to demand a vocation "find your purpose" or to load a discovered vector with obligations. *Minimal counter-experience.* Here the invariant is itself the form the counter-experience strengthens: to help directedness take hold — to resonate in the body, to sound in contact, to find a word, to link with a small action in its direction — so that the vector gains a path to repetition. *Frequent clusters / where it occurs.* Noetic family; an integrative marker. Often with the presence of meaning (P-NO1), restored agency (P-AG3), and the witnessing "I" as a sign of a collected, stable assembly.

H.4. From invariant to cluster

A single invariant is rarely a complete formulation. What becomes clinically significant is the cluster — several forms that together organize the current R(t) and support one another. A folded future makes the world cramped, a cramped world drains action of meaning, halted action confirms the no-way-out — and the cluster holds itself by the same recursion described in Chapter 3.

This is why the atlas is read not as a list of labels but as a set of directions of hearing: having heard one form, one asks which other forms hold beside it and what assembly they form together. In a working formulation, three to five load-bearing invariants are usually enough — the bundle that actually holds the assembly now. Stable, frequently recurring clusters unfold into configuration prototypes (Appendix I); but a prototype is not an obligatory frame: sometimes reality is organized by one or two vivid invariants, and the formulation stays at the level of a cluster.

The connection between the appendices is simple. H answers the question "which form sounds." I shows into which recognizable assemblies these forms combine. Chapter 10 gives the principle holding both: to hear not only what the client says, but the form of reality within which his words become true — and not to confuse the map of the form with the person himself.

Appendix I. Configuration Families and CCP Prototypes

A working support for Chapter 10. Ten prototypes, five families, the vertical stability axis O1–O5.

I.1. How to use this appendix

This appendix unfolds what Chapter 10 only names: ten prototypical configurations (CCP), grouped for convenience into five families, and the vertical stability axis O1–O5. Each prototype is given as a card — a working map of reading, not a passport of a disorder.

Before using the cards, one must hold four defenses, without which the appendix immediately turns into what all of Chapter 10 warns against:

- A CCP is not a diagnosis. It is a map of the organization of experience active now, not a category to which a person belongs. One cannot "have" a CCP the way one has a diagnosis.
- A family is not a type of person. The five families exist only for navigation among the ten names. They are not diagnoses, not new configurations, and not a theoretical level.
- An O-level is not a label of severity. The axis O1–O5 is read as the integrative stability and the risk of disorganization of the current assembly, not as a scale of the severity of a personality.
- A card helps formulate a hypothesis, it does not replace clinical reading. If a card does not make the therapist more attentive to the living material, it should be set aside.

Each card answers not the question "what type of client is this" but the question: which organization of experience is active now, what it does with reality, where the veto most often arises, what is usually premature, and which minimal different experience can begin a shift. The fields "typical dominant constraint" and "what is often premature" are frequent candidates, not prescriptions: the veto is determined by triangulation on the concrete material (Appendix C), not by the name of the configuration.

I.2. The five families of configurations

Ten names are hard to hold in mind at once, so — and only for this — they are grouped into five families. The families need not be equal in size and make no claim to completeness.

1. **Temporal-transitional (CCP-1, 2, 10).** Configurations in which time is disordered — the link between "then," "now," and "later." Compression of the future, intrusion of the past, frozen transition. The common question of reading: what has happened to the temporal structure of experience.
2. **Self-protective (CCP-3, 4).** The assembly is organized around the defense of the self — from an unbearable uncertainty (defensive clarity) or from a destroying visibility (shame organization of the self). The common question: what exactly the self defends against, and at what cost.
3. **Intersubjective-attachment (CCP-5, 9).** Both forms are about how the other is disordered: there is too much of him, to the point of inseparability (attachment without differentiation), or there is none of him at all, the field has emptied (intersubjective absence). The common question: how the other is present or absent.
4. **Agentic-active (CCP-6, 7).** Both are about a disorder of action: there is none, "I can" has vanished (collapse of agency), or there is, but it bypasses meaning, discharges before becoming experience (action without symbolization). The common question: how action is built and whether it passes through the subject and through meaning.
5. **Noetic-semantic (CCP-8).** In this family there is so far one prototype — noetic overload — and this is normal: a family solves the task of orientation, not of symmetry. Other noetic forms (collapse of meaning, thinning, loss of directedness) more often appear as invariants within different configurations; overload is singled out specifically because it forms a stable, self-standing configurational logic.

I.3. The ten CCP prototypes

CCP-1. Compression of the future. *Brief logic.* The future is folded to the almost-present: tomorrow and next year are experienced as one bearing-down thing in which there is no air to breathe. The future is not empty — it has collapsed, and no room is left in it for anything to unfold. *Phenomenological cluster.* Folded time (temporal); the world narrowed to the bearing-down (world); action halted — "what's the point of planning" (agentic); affect colored by no-way-out (affective). The cluster holds itself: a cramped world drains action of meaning, halted action confirms the no-way-out, the no-way-out folds time still further. *How it sounds in the session.* "I have no future," but on being asked about plans the very space in which a plan could fit narrows. Talk of tomorrow and of next year goes without difference of scale. Bodily — constriction, lack of air at the thought of "later." *Typical dominant constraint.* Often the narrative N(t) or predictive activity Pσ, when "nothing ahead" works as anticipatory knowledge; sometimes the life-world Λ, if the future is really blocked by external conditions. *What is often premature.* Planning, goal-setting, "small steps" — there is nowhere to put a plan while the space of the future is compressed. Reassurance "it will work out" bounces off. *Minimal counter-experience.* A small experience that there is a gap between "now" and "later": one experience in which the future unfolds, for a second, by at least a step — not a plan, but a sense that time again has depth. *Frequent reading error.* To hear the content "no future" and start building a future, without hearing that the very form of time is folded. To confuse it with depressive hopelessness as a theme rather than as a temporal form. *Not a diagnosis.* The configuration may be active today and inactive tomorrow; it is read, not assigned.

CCP-2. Intrusion of the past. *Brief logic.* The past has not passed — it lasts in the present as something happening now. "Then" is not closed and automatically organizes "now"; the reaction in the present is clearly larger than the current event. *Phenomenological cluster.* The past intrudes into the present (temporal); a developmental calibration in which today is experienced by the measure of a long-ago scene; the affect of the long-ago situation is active here; sometimes the body reacts to the current as to the former threat. *How it sounds in the session.* The reaction is disproportionate to the occasion; today's person or situation is met by the measure of a long-ago one. The client may be aware of it — "I understand he's not my father" — and still react as to a father. *Typical dominant constraint.* Often developmental calibration D_cal; with falling coherence on approaching the material — the thresholds Θ; the body B(t), if the intrusion goes bodily. *What is often premature.* Work only with the current event — it does not reach what organizes the reaction. Strong confrontation with the "irrationality" of the reaction strengthens the defense. *Minimal counter-experience.* A small experience of distinguishing "then" and "now": a moment in which the present is experienced as the present, not as a repetition. Often through the body and field, not through explanation. *Frequent reading error.* To take the intrusion of the past for an actual conflict and work with today's content; or to confuse it with CCP-1 — but there the future is disordered, here the past lasts. *Not a diagnosis.* This is a form of time active in the moment, not a property of the personality.

CCP-3. Defensive clarity. *Brief logic.* Reality is assembled with a deceptive sharpness in which everything is "clear." This clarity is not cognition but a defense: it closes off an unbearable uncertainty. Clarity here serves not truth but the stability of the assembly. *Phenomenological cluster.* The world is assembled as finally understood (world); novelty bounces off, turning into confirmation of the known (low permeability); the affect of uncertainty is displaced; the narrative is sealed — "there's nothing to explore here, it's just a fact." *How it sounds in the session.* Quick final formulations, an even confident tone, "it's all clear." Curiosity about one's own experience is absent; the question "could it be otherwise" meets not anger but a closing-down. *Typical dominant constraint.* Often the defensively closed Cα mode; the narrative N(t) absorbing the new into a ready schema; sometimes the thresholds Θ, if behind the clarity is a fear of disintegration under uncertainty. *What is often premature.* Confrontation of the clarity, demonstration of contradictions, "have you not thought that..." — all this is read as an encroachment and strengthens the closure. Arguing with content is useless: the problem is not in the belief but in the function of the clarity. *Minimal counter-experience.* A small experience of bearable uncertainty: a moment in which "I don't know" does not bring things down but turns out bearable in a safe field. Not a destruction of the clarity, but a trial that one can live for a second without it. *Frequent reading error.* To take defensive clarity for genuine understanding and the client's "agreement" — and to celebrate an integration that is not there; or to take the closure for intellectualization as a trait. *Not a diagnosis.* Clarity here is the work of the assembly in the moment, not a type of the person's thinking.

CCP-4. Shame organization of the self. *Brief logic.* A configuration in which the self is organized around the experience of a destroying visibility: to be seen means to be appraised, and to be appraised means to be found wanting. Reality is assembled so that the other's gaze is read in advance as condemning, and the system spends its forces on becoming smaller, less noticeable, more flawless. Shame here is not an emotion among emotions but a form that gives weight to all the rest of experience. *Phenomenological cluster.* Load-bearing invariants (not the whole list — a recognizable bundle of four to six): visibility is experienced as a threat ("I am seen — so I am appraised"); the self is fragile, organized around a defect that cannot be shown; the other is present as an appraising gaze (intersubjective invariant); action contracts to the avoidance of exposure — not to present, not to stick out (agentic); the affect is colored by anticipatory shame, even before real contact. *How it sounds in the session.* The client apologizes for each of his manifestations, awaits appraisal in advance, contracts under a gaze. Bodily — dropped shoulders, averted gaze, the voice quieter toward the end of the phrase. In the field — a heightened sensitivity to the slightest signal of disapproval, a tendency to read the therapist's neutral face as condemning. Behaviorally — presents himself in doses, checks the reaction before opening a little more. *Typical dominant constraint.* Not one forever — frequent candidates worth checking by triangulation (Appendix C): the field S(t), when the current contact with the therapist itself is not yet lived as safe for visibility; developmental calibration D_cal, when today's gaze is read by the measure of a long-ago scene of humiliation; the high reality weight of shame (RW3–RW4), when "I am shameful" is not a belief but a self-sealed reality; the thresholds Θ, when approaching the shame material brings down coherence. *What is often premature.* Direct naming of shame ("it seems you feel very ashamed") in a field that has not yet lived safety of visibility. Praise and encouragement — they strengthen the exposure and are often read as one more appraisal. Work with early shame scenes before visibility in the room has become bearable. Any exposure task "present yourself to the world," demanding action from a system that has not yet lived safety of visibility even here. *Minimal counter-experience.* The most important field of the card. For CCP-4 this is an experience of a small visibility without added shame: a moment in which the client is seen — and not appraised, not comforted too quickly, not corrected. Not a naming of shame, but a living-through that here one can be seen and not judged. Before this — a tuning of the field: a restoration of contact, the experience that in the room one is not appraised. If even a small visibility is so far impossible, the question is asked again, one step lower: what must become possible earlier so that even a minimal experience of being seen becomes bearable. *Frequent reading error.* To take the shame organization for low self-esteem, avoidance, resistance, or narcissistic vulnerability — and to work with the label instead of the form. But the costliest error is different and is described in the opening of Chapter 11: to hear the shame form rightly and stop at it too early, without checking whether the life-world Λ holds the veto. If the client is systematically humiliated by a real environment — a boss, a family, an unsafe contract — then the dominant constraint now is not in the shame and not in the therapy field but in Λ, and inner work with shame without a change of conditions is premature, and at times sounds like a subtle accusation: "you ought to experience differently what is objectively destroying you." A precise form is not a reason to stop asking what else holds the situation. *Not a diagnosis.* This configuration may be active in the moment and does not describe the whole person. The same client in another field, in another Cα mode, may assemble differently. CCP-4 is a map of the current assembly, not a property of the personality; it is read, not assigned. If this map does not make the therapist more attentive to the living material, it should be set aside.

CCP-5. Attachment without differentiation. *Brief logic.* The other is needed to the point of inseparability: to be oneself beside him is impossible, because separateness is experienced as a threat to the bond or as abandonment. Self and other are assembled into one, and the boundary between them does not hold. *Phenomenological cluster.* The other is needed to the point of merging (intersubjective); the self loses its contours beside the other (self); action is subordinated to holding the bond (agentic); the affect of anxiety at any sign of separateness. *How it sounds in the session.* A strong reaction to pauses, breaks, the end of the session; a quick reading of the therapist's state and an adjustment to it; difficulty naming one's own desire distinct from the other's. In the field — a pressure of merging, a thinness at any differentiation. *Typical dominant constraint.* Often the field S(t), when separation in contact itself is un-integrable; developmental calibration D_cal, if merging is a long-ago form; the thresholds Θ on approaching the experience of separateness. *What is often premature.* Encouragement of autonomy, "you need to learn to be more independent," work toward separation before the bond is lived as reliable. Premature differentiation is read as abandonment. *Minimal counter-experience.* A small experience of separateness without loss of the bond: a moment in which the client differs a little, disagrees a little — and the bond does not tear. That one can be oneself and stay together. *Frequent reading error.* To take attachment without differentiation for a "dependent disorder" as a trait; or to confuse it with CCP-9 — but there the other is not present at all, here there is too much of the other. *Not a diagnosis.* This is a form of the other's presence in the current assembly, not a personality type.

CCP-6. Collapse of agency. *Brief logic.* "I can" has vanished: action does not come from the subject but either does not begin or happens to me. Will is not experienced as one's own; between intention and action there is a void. *Phenomenological cluster.* Action does not come from me (agentic); the self is passive, undergoes (self); the future has no vector, because there is no one to act in it; an affect of powerlessness or numbness. *How it sounds in the session.* "I can't make myself," "it doesn't get done by itself," describing one's own life in the passive voice. Not laziness and not sabotage — an absence of the experience of outgoing action. *Typical dominant constraint.* Often the body B(t) under deep exhaustion or depressive retardation; the life-world Λ, if the environment really deprives one of agency; sometimes developmental calibration D_cal. *What is often premature.* Activating tasks, "just start small," action plans — they require an agency that is not there now, and each unfulfilled step confirms the powerlessness. *Minimal counter-experience.* A small experience of outgoing action: a micro-movement experienced as "I did this" — not a result, but a return of authorship in the smallest thing. *Frequent reading error.* To take the collapse of agency for low motivation, laziness, or resistance; not to check the body and the environment, where the veto most often holds. *Not a diagnosis.* This is a state of agency in the moment, not a characteristic of the person's will.

CCP-7. Action without symbolization. *Brief logic.* Action exists, but it does not pass through meaning: it discharges before becoming experience. The impulse passes into the deed, bypassing symbolic processing — and so it does not learn from itself and does not nourish. *Phenomenological cluster.* Action bypasses meaning (agentic + noetic); affect discharges in the deed rather than being experienced; the narrative of the action is poor — "I just did it"; a weak link between the done and the lived. *How it sounds in the session.* Impulsive deeds, acting-out, difficulty stopping and feeling what stands behind the action. Telling of events without an inner layer; a repetition of the same discharges. *Typical dominant constraint.* Often the thresholds Θ, if symbolization brings down coherence; the body B(t) under high activation; sometimes the narrative N(t), when there is no language for the experience. *What is often premature.* Interpretation of the meaning of the deed, "what did you really feel" — the symbolic layer is not yet available, and the question hangs or produces a pseudo-answer. A ban on action without an alternative strengthens the discharge. *Minimal counter-experience.* A small experience of a pause between impulse and action, in which at least some experience manages to appear: a moment when between "I wanted to" and "I did" a thin layer of feeling arises. *Frequent reading error.* To take the discharge for "expression of emotion" and encourage it; or to moralize the deeds instead of reading the form in which action bypasses meaning. *Not a diagnosis.* This is a form of the link between action and meaning in the moment, not impulsivity as a trait.

CCP-8. Noetic overload. *Brief logic.* There is not too little meaning but unbearably much: everything is significant at once. Each detail is loaded with meaning, nothing can be neutral or background, and the system is overloaded by an excess of meaning, not by its absence. *Phenomenological cluster.* A hypertrophy of salience — salience is distributed onto everything (salience); meaning has grown to overload (noetic); the world is excessively significant in every detail (world); an affect of tense captivation; sometimes a disturbance of the filter of the relevant. *How it sounds in the session.* Everything is connected with everything, any detail pulls a chain of meanings, it is hard to single out the main thing. Speech is saturated, branching; a fatigue from the impossibility of resting from meaning. May approach aberrant salience — here it is important to read the O vertical. *Typical dominant constraint.* Often the thresholds Θ and coherence; at O4–O5 or a shift toward them — a risk of disorganization where salience becomes aberrant (see I.4 and the boundary of safety). Sometimes the body B(t) — an overload of regulation. *What is often premature.* Deepening of meanings, a search for "one more meaning" — this adds to the overload. Cognitive work on distinguishing the important from the background is premature while the overall load is not lowered. *Minimal counter-experience.* A small experience of the neutral: a moment in which something can be simply background, not loaded with meaning. A rest from meaning, not a new meaning. *Frequent reading error.* To take the overload for a richness of associations or intellectual liveliness; to miss the O vertical and not notice a shift toward O4–O5, where specialized assessment is needed. *Not a diagnosis.* This is a form of the work of meaning in the moment; at signs of disorganization safety comes first, not reading the configuration.

CCP-9. Intersubjective absence. *Brief logic.* The other is not present as alive: the field has emptied of people. People are there physically but are not experienced as real presences; contact goes through glass. This is not loneliness as a feeling, but a form in which the other has lost liveness. *Phenomenological cluster.* The other is lifeless, the field has emptied (intersubjective); the self in isolation, sometimes derealized (self); affect is blunted, the world bleached (affective); the meaning of contact is thinned.

How it sounds in the session. Describing relationships without liveness, "as if behind glass," difficulty feeling the therapist as real. In the field — a sense that contact does not form, despite formally correct interaction. The therapist may feel "invisible" or interchangeable. *Typical dominant constraint.* Often the field S(t), when living contact itself is un-integrable; the thresholds Θ under derealization; the body B(t), if the absence goes through blunting; sometimes the O-level under marked dissociation. *What is often premature.* Emotionally saturated interventions, calls to closeness, "let's stay in contact" — the field does not withstand a living presence, and pressing strengthens the withdrawal behind glass. *Minimal counter-experience.* A small experience of the other's living presence without overload: a brief moment in which the therapist is experienced as real and this is bearable. A dose of liveness the field is able to let through. *Frequent reading error.* To take the absence for coldness, avoidance, or a "schizoid trait"; or to confuse it with CCP-5 — but there the other is too much, here he is not there at all. *Not a diagnosis.* This is a form of the other's presence in the current assembly, not a property of the personality.

CCP-10. Frozen transition. *Brief logic.* The person is stuck between the old organization and a new one: neither holds. The former form no longer assembles reality, the new has not yet assembled, and the system hangs in the interval, where there is support neither in the old nor in the new. *Phenomenological cluster.* The transitional link of time is disordered — between "who I was" and "who I am becoming" (temporal); the self without a stable form (self); action is irresolute, because there is nothing to act from; an affect of suspension, sometimes the anxiety of supportlessness. *How it sounds in the session.* "I'm no longer the one I was, but I haven't become another," "everything is hung up," an impossibility of either returning or moving. Not a crisis of choice, but an absence of a support from which a choice could be made. *Typical dominant constraint.* Often the thresholds Θ — coherence falls in the interval; the field S(t) as a temporary support; sometimes the narrative N(t), if there is no language for the transition. *What is often premature.* Pushing toward a decision, "it's time to move on," help in choosing a new form — the transition cannot be hurried, and pressing strengthens the supportlessness. A return to the old form does not work either: it no longer holds. *Minimal counter-experience.* A small experience of support in the interval itself: a moment in which the suspension is bearable, and the field holds, while the new form has not yet assembled. Not an acceleration of the transition, but a bearability of its middle. *Frequent reading error.* To take the frozen transition for irresoluteness as a trait or for resistance to change; to force movement where what is needed is support in the interval. *Not a diagnosis.* This is a transitional state of the assembly, by definition temporary.

I.4. The vertical axis O1–O5: the stability of the assembly

The horizontal (which form is assembled) and the vertical (how stably it holds) are read together. Invariants, clusters, and configurations answer the question which form is active. The axis O1–O5 answers another: how stably the assembly itself holds under the current load — whether it will stay whole under pressure or begin to fall apart. This is an axis of integrative stability and of the risk of disorganization, not a scale of severity and not an appraisal of the person; like everything in Chapter 10, it pertains to the moment.

- **O1 — stable organization.** R(t) is coherent; self, time, other, and action are held; the system withstands novelty and contradiction without disintegration.
- **O2 — traumatically fragile.** Coherence usually holds but falls under certain triggers, affects, or relational loads; outside them it looks stable.
- **O3 — borderline-unstable.** The assembly switches quickly; the other, the field, and reality weight sharply change the availability of self and action from session to session and within a session.
- **O4 — dissociatively fragmented.** The coherence of self, memory, body, or agency may fall apart into states that hold together poorly.
- **O5 — psychotically disorganizing.** The field of shared reality is disturbed; unusual connections, aberrant salience, or disturbances of reality testing begin to organize R(t).

The clinical sense of the axis is in the permissible load. The less stable the assembly, the lower the permissible integration load and the more safety, specialized assessment, and supervision matter. The same configuration at different O-levels is, in essence, different clinical situations under one name.

How the axis modifies a configuration: the example of CCP-4. The shame organization of the self looks and works differently depending on the stability of the assembly:

- CCP-4 at O1 — shame is active, but the self withstands visibility; the counter-experience of small visibility is bearable and takes hold.
- CCP-4 at O2 — shame is sharply activated by triggers, but outside them coherence holds; work is possible with attention to the trigger zones.
- CCP-4 at O3 — shame may quickly switch the state of self and the relationship; the same intervention now lands, now brings things down, and the pace is dictated by the instability.
- CCP-4 at O4 — shame is linked with dissociative breaks, ruptures of self and body; a counter-experience useful at O1 may here fragment.
- CCP-4 at O5 — shame enters a disorganizing field of reality; what comes first is not work with the configuration but specialized assessment and safety.

The same principle applies to any CCP: the vertical says what load work with this form will withstand now. A detailed mapping of the levels with indicators is in development; for practice it matters most to read the axis as stability and the risk of disorganization, not as a label of severity, and to remember that it too is about the moment.

End of Appendix I.

Appendix J. The School Compatibility Matrix

A working support for Chapter 12. A brief map of the translation of DDSRF concepts into already-existing clinical languages.

J.1. Why this matrix

This matrix is not an encyclopedia of psychotherapeutic schools. It does not retell their theory, does not assess their completeness, and does not claim that DDSRF "gives" them what they lack. Its task is more modest: to show how the concepts of DDSRF can be used as a grammar of case formulation, sequence, and integrability within different clinical languages.

Through all ten cards runs one thing. Each school remains itself, with its own techniques and its own criteria of rightness. DDSRF adds a common language for the layer where the schools usually diverge — for the reading of the moment: what is assembled now, which mode, which weight, what holds the veto, what must become possible earlier. This is what makes it translatable, not competing.

The card format has four fields: the native language of the school, the translation into DDSRF, what DDSRF does not assert, the supervision question. There are ten cards. If truly needed, other approaches may be added by the same principle — but the matrix deliberately does not sprawl: its value is in brevity and in the discipline of the four fields.

J.2. The ten school cards

Psychoanalysis and psychodynamic therapy. *Native language of the school.* Transference, countertransference, interpretation, the unconscious, defense, containment, the choice of the moment, symbolization. *Translation into DDSRF.* S(t) as the field of the other, the therapist's counter-load, the Cα mode, the dominant constraint, sequence; "premature interpretation" acquires an operational sense — an intervention into the defensively closed mode. *What DDSRF does not assert.* DDSRF replaces neither transference nor work with the unconscious, history, deep symbolization. Analytic listening remains analytic listening. *Supervision question.* Does the interpretation land in the field now — or add a load that S(t) does not withstand?

Relational and Gestalt approaches. *Native language of the school.* Contact, boundary, field, meeting, here-and-now, awareness, interruption of contact. *Translation into DDSRF.* S(t), the integrative capacity of the field, the Cα mode, the minimal counter-experience; an interruption of contact is read as an event in the field, not only in the client. *What DDSRF does not assert.* DDSRF does not replace living contact with a grammar and does not reduce the meeting to a schema. It is an instrument for reading the moment, not a way to live it. *Supervision question.* What is happening to novelty in the field of contact now — does it land, bounce off, or fragment?

CBT and process-based CBT. *Native language of the school.* Beliefs, schemas, cognitive shifts, behavioral experiments, exposure, processes of change. *Translation into DDSRF.* Reality weight (RW), predictive activity Pσ, the zone of fit of load and capacity, the minimal counter-experience. *What DDSRF does not assert.* DDSRF does not assert that cognitive work is superficial. It asserts that a cognitive change becomes clinically strong when the new content gains reality weight. *Supervision question.* Has this cognitive change already become a lived reality — or has it stayed at RW0–RW1?

ACT. *Native language of the school.* Defusion, acceptance, values, psychological flexibility, committed action, the six core processes. *Translation into DDSRF.* RW, noetic invariants, agency, the minimal counter-experience; flexibility as the availability of several assemblies, rather than one correct one. *What DDSRF does not assert.* DDSRF does not replace the model of psychological flexibility and does not dictate the content of values. Flexibility remains flexibility, values remain the client's. *Supervision question.* Is the value-action integrable now — or premature relative to the Cα mode, RW, and the dominant constraint?

DBT. *Native language of the school.* Regulation, skills, the dialectic of acceptance and change, crisis safety, validation. *Translation into DDSRF.* The body B(t), the coherence thresholds Θ, the fragmenting and stabilizing

$C\alpha$ modes, integrative capacity; stabilization as a building-up of capacity, not "insufficient therapy." *What DDSRF does not assert.* DDSRF does not replace skills training, crisis protocols, and safety work. Safety stands above any logic of reading the moment. *Supervision question.* Is transformation needed now — or first a restoration of coherence and capacity?

CFT. *Native language of the school.* Shame, self-criticism, threat, the soothing system, compassion, the three motivational systems. *Translation into DDSRF.* The RW of shame, S(t), the $P\sigma$ of threat, the minimal experience of safe visibility; the shame organization as an assembly, not a "personality trait." *What DDSRF does not assert.* DDSRF does not reduce compassion to a technique for lowering shame and does not replace the CFT model of motivational systems. *Supervision question.* Does the compassionate intervention land as a new possibility — or is it experienced as appraisal, praise, pressure?

EMDR and phase-based trauma therapy. *Native language of the school.* The window of tolerance, stabilization, processing, titration, dual attention, traumatic memory, the phase structure. *Translation into DDSRF.* The thresholds Θ, the body B(t), reality weight, developmental calibration D_cal, the principle of sequence, the minimal counter-experience; the window of tolerance as a particular case of the zone of fit in bodily-affective regulation. *What DDSRF does not assert.* DDSRF does not replace specialized trauma therapy and does not cancel the phase discipline of safety. Stabilization is work, not waiting. *Supervision question.* Is the processing now within the zone of fit — or does it exceed coherence and go beyond the window?

Somatic approaches. *Native language of the school.* The body, interoception, autonomic regulation, grounding, bodily memory, polyvagal states. *Translation into DDSRF.* B(t), Θ, the Load–Capacity–Field Grid (Appendix E), the bodily or regulatory trace of the counter-experience (M4 in Appendix F). *What DDSRF does not assert.* DDSRF does not assert that the body explains everything. The body is one of the layers of the assembly, which often holds veto power, but not the only one. *Supervision question.* Does the bodily work increase capacity now — or become a new load the assembly does not integrate?

Systemic and family therapy. *Native language of the school.* Circularity, patterns of interaction, the family system, context, boundaries, hypothesizing. *Translation into DDSRF.* S(t), the life-world Λ, the recursivity of the assembly from R(t) to R(t+1), the dominant constraint in the field or the life-world. *What DDSRF does not assert.* DDSRF does not reduce the system to the individual psyche and does not replace systemic thinking with an individual formulation. *Supervision question.* Is what looks like an inner problem not being supported right now by a real system of relationships or by the life-world?

Existential and humanistic therapy. *Native language of the school.* Meaning, freedom, choice, presence, authenticity, meeting, responsibility. *Translation into DDSRF.* Noetic invariants, agency, S(t), the reality weight of meaning, the minimal counter-experience. *What DDSRF does not assert.* DDSRF does not dictate the content of meaning and does not replace the living meeting with a grammar. The content remains the person's; the model is about the conditions in which it can become livable. *Supervision question.* Does the conversation about meaning open a livable possibility now — or become too high a noetic load?

J.3. How to use the matrix in supervision

The matrix is needed not to translate the client from one school into DDSRF. It is needed so that a therapist of his own school can ask: what does my school see well now, what may it not see, and what language of DDSRF helps to check this?

Useful supervision questions when working with the matrix:

- Which language of my school is leading the case formulation now?
- What does this language see well — which layer of the assembly is transparent in it?
- What may it not see — which layer stays beyond its usual focus?
- Where does DDSRF help check the fit of an intervention, reality weight, the $C\alpha$ mode, the dominant constraint, or sequence?
- Have I begun to use DDSRF as a language of superiority over my own school — or as a way to bypass its discipline?

Special attention is worth giving to the fifth question. The matrix easily turns into an instrument of subtle devaluation of other schools — "we translate you into our language, and now it's clearer to you." This contradicts the very logic of DDSRF as a grammar. The translation is honest when it works in both directions: the concepts of DDSRF are translatable into the language of the school, and the language of the school remains clinically sovereign.

Final formula. The compatibility of DDSRF with the schools is tested not by how beautifully its concepts translate, but by whether this translation helps the therapist work more precisely within his own clinical tradition. If it translates but does not help — the translation has failed, and the matrix in that row needs refining. If it helps without violating the discipline of the school — the matrix has done its work.

End of Appendix J.

Appendix K. The Epistemic and Normative Register

A working support for Chapter 12.

Why this register

The statements of DDSRF are not equal in force. Some are a working notation, a way of speaking; others an observation distinguishable in the material; still others a so-far-unproven hypothesis; and yet others a clinical obligation that does not wait for proofs. To present them with the same confidence is to mislead the reader. The register gives each statement two independent coordinates: how far we know it (epistemic status, ES) and how far it obliges (normative status, NS). This is the same discipline that holds Chapter 12: the maturity of the model lies not in an even confidence but in knowing the force of each of its own statements.

The register is a working instrument, not a philosophical declaration. It is used when one needs to check whether a convenient notation is passing itself off as a fact and whether a necessary action is being postponed until a mechanism is proven. This is the same discipline of revisability that in Chapter 11 was applied to the clinical formulation; here it is applied to the statements of DDSRF itself.

Axis 1. Epistemic status: ES0–ES5

The scale answers one question: how reliably we know what we assert.

- **ES0 — conceptual frame.** A way of speaking, a notation, not a proven mechanism. The notation R(t), the operator Cα as a designation of the assembly. To call R(t) a notation is not to weaken the theory but to keep it from passing off a convenient notation as a discovery.

- **ES1 — phenomenological observation.** A descriptive structure of experience, distinguishable in the material. Invariants as forms of experience. The maturity of a particular invariant may at that differ: some are long described and easily recognized, others recently proposed.
- **ES2 — clinical heuristic.** A working distinction, useful at the bedside but not proven as an entity. The dominant constraint, the Cα modes, the levels of reality weight. These are instruments of reading, not measured quantities.
- **ES3 — mechanistic hypothesis.** A plausible M-description requiring testing: the links of the assembly with the body, prediction, memory. It sounds like hard science and for that very reason most often risks an overstatement of status.
- **ES4 — testable hypothesis.** What can and should be put under an empirical test: ICAE, the principle of sequence, the inter-rater agreement of recognition, the predictive usefulness of the formulation.
- **ES5 — confirmed statement.** Here it must be said honestly: in the current version the new constructs of DDSRF should almost never claim this status. Part of the background clinical and scientific premises on which the model rests has high external support, but the DDSRF-specific statements are for now obliged to remain more cautious.

The scale guards against inflation of status — a characteristic failure of young theories, when a successful notation like $R(t) = C\alpha[\ldots]$ begins to sound like a measured quantity, and the metaphor of the assembly operator like a mechanism discovered in the brain. An explicit mark keeps the theory's promises within what it can actually present. For a two-domain model this is especially important: M-descriptions sound temptingly like hard science, and it is they that are most often threatened with overstatement.

Axis 2. Normative status: NS0–NS3

The scale answers a different question: how far a statement obliges to action. Epistemic status and normative status are different axes. A theoretical proposition may be no more than a notation and prescribe nothing; a clinical requirement may be obligatory without being a proven mechanism.

- **NS0 — no prescription.** A purely descriptive proposition. Dictates nothing to behavior.
- **NS1 — clinical caution.** A reason to be more attentive, no more.
- **NS2 — strong recommendation.** To depart from it is worth doing only with a clear ground.
- **NS3 — boundary of safety.** A situation where specialized help is required and where the ordinary logic of the model steps back. The obligation here does not wait for theoretical proof.

The two axes read together

The habit of reading a statement along both axes at once quickly becomes automatic. Each coordinate answers its own question: how far we know it — and how far it obliges.

Statement	ES	NS
The notation R(t) = Cα[...] as a way of speaking about the assembly	ES0	NS0
"Reality weight is held by several layers"	ES2	NS0
"At high RW one contradicting experience is usually not enough unless it passes through body, field, narrative, and action"	ES2	NS2
"Do not force traumatic material under falling coherence"	ES2–4	NS2
"At signs of psychotic disorganization a psychiatric assessment is needed"	any	NS3

Two typical errors arise precisely from confusing the axes: to turn a beautiful theoretical notation into an obligatory rule — or, conversely, to postpone a necessary action until the mechanism is proven. Safety does not wait for proofs; notation does not dictate behavior.

The rule of five registers

For the register to work in living speech and in supervision, it is useful not to mix five different things that in a text easily sound equally confident:

1. A conceptual frame — notation and a way of speaking (ES0).

2. A clinical heuristic — a working distinction at the bedside (ES2).
3. A hypothesis — plausible but untested (ES3).
4. A testable statement — what can be put under a test (ES4).
5. A clinical-ethical prescription — an obligation, including the boundary of safety (the normative axis, up to NS3).

The first four are about knowledge. The fifth is about obligation. To hold them apart means not to pass off a frame as a fact, a hypothesis as established, or a recommendation as a notation. This is the epistemic discipline of DDSRF applied to itself.

End of Appendix K.

End of the DDSRF Method Atlas (Appendices A–K).

About the Author

Shiraz Mamedov is a psychologist and the author of the DDSRF model. His work centers on case formulation, sequence, integrability, and the conditions under which a clinical intervention becomes clinically usable. The model is addressed to practicing clinicians, supervisors, teachers, and researchers across therapeutic orientations.

www.ingramcontent.com/pod-product-compliance
Lightning Source LLC
LaVergne TN
LVHW022207200926
848481LV00006B/1883
* 9 7 9 8 9 9 6 5 1 5 5 0 9 *